Serial Dissections
of the
Human Brain

Serial Dissections of the Human Brain

Carlton G. Smith, M.D., Ph.D.

Professor Emeritus of Anatomy
University of Toronto Faculty of
Medicine

Visiting Professor of Anatomy
Uniformed Services University of the Health Sciences
Bethesda

Urban & Schwarzenberg · Baltimore–Munich 1981

Urban & Schwarzenberg, Inc.
7 E. Redwood Street
Baltimore, Maryland 21202
USA

Urban & Schwarzenberg
Pettenkoferstrasse 18
D-8000 München 2
Germany

Printed in the United States of America

Library of Congress Cataloging in Publication Data

Smith, Carlton George.
   Serial dissections of the human brain.

   Includes index.
   1. Brain—Anatomy—Atlases. 2. Human dissection—Atlases. I. Title. [DNLM:
1. Brain—Anatomy and histology—Atlases.
2. Dissection—Atlases. WL 17 S644s]
QM455.S64   611′.81   81-2540
ISBN 0-8067-1811-0   AACR2

ISBN 0-8067-1811-0 Baltimore

ISBN 3-541-71811-0 Munich

Contents

Preface

The purpose of this atlas is twofold; to make available photographs of 1) serial dissections of the cerebral hemisphere and the cerebellum and 2) the major pathways of the brain stem.

This work is not intended to be a substitute for textbooks. The photographs herein supplement textbook descriptions of the cell masses and fiber bundles of the brain by visualizing them in three dimensions. The atlas is designed to be useful to all who have an interest in the mechanisms of the brain. This includes not only medical and dental students, but also those in the allied health sciences and psychology—in short, all students in the neuroscience field.

Serial dissections of the "appendages" of the brain stem, and isolation of the sensory and motor pathways within the brain stem are special features of this work. All the dissections were prepared and personally photographed by the author to ensure that important parts were clearly delineated. To avoid obscuring detail with labels, almost all of the labeling is confined to line drawings made from tracings of the photographs. These drawings also draw attention to significant features of the dissections. Because the relationships of pathways are easily seen in the photographs, the pathologist may find them to be useful for reference in correlating lesions and clinical findings.

In addition to serving as an aid to understanding textbook descriptions of the structure of the brain, this atlas will be of assistance to those who may have the opportunity to dissect a brain. To that end, some basic features of techniques of brain dissection that the author has found helpful, are included.

It is with pleasure that I acknowledge my indebtedness to Dr. Keith L. Moore, Chairman of the Department of Anatomy, University of Toronto. His encouragement and assistance are much appreciated. In addition, I am indebted to my wife, Marguerite (Harland) Smith, for her valuable contributions to all phases of this work.

Toronto, *Spring 1981*

CARLTON G. SMITH

Introduction

The dissections prepared for this atlas reveal all the major pathways that a skilled dissector is able to isolate. Therefore, the photographs and accompanying labeled drawings will serve as a substitute for the instructional value of dissection for those who lack the opportunity to dissect the brain. If dissecting facilities are available, this atlas will serve as a useful guide in achieving adequate preparations.

The following precautions and suggestions will assist the would-be dissector and make the undertaking more rewarding. It is essential that the brain be well fixed by immersion in 10% formaldehyde at the time of autopsy and then left for at least one month. Formaldehyde fixation is preferable to other fixatives because it toughens the nerve fibers without making them brittle. With a well-hardened brain, cleavage planes can be opened up in the core of the white matter of both the cerebral hemisphere and the cerebellum, where fibers of major pathways are aggregated into large, compact bundles. A dissecting probe with a slender, smooth, bent tip is an indispensable instrument for seeking a cleavage plane. It is used as a wedge and, being smooth, can be moved along a cleavage plane to follow fibers to their termination.

In carrying out a progressive dissection of the brain, it is necessary to remove each fiber bundle or layer of fibers as it is encountered. To do this, fibers are stripped away a few at a time until the probe encounters fibers coursing in a different direction. This is an indication that another pathway has been uncovered. An example of such a finding is seen in Figures 5 and 6, where the removal of the superior longitudinal fasciculus exposes the fiber layer called the corona radiata.

The isolation of the large bundles of fibers of the cerebral hemisphere is relatively easy, but following the smaller bundles of the brain stem is a challenge. Here the first step is to remove the thin, paint-like, rubbery, external, limiting layer of neuroglia by slipping a dissecting needle under it and peeling it away. This will reveal the fibers of the pathways that lie on its surface. These are unlike the fiber bundles of the cerebral hemisphere that lie deep to a superficial layer of gray matter. A bent pin serves as a useful miniature probe in isolating one of these fiber bundles within the brain stem.

To assist the dissector in tracing the relatively small fiber bundles along the length of the brain stem, reference can be made to the cross-sections where their positions and the form of their cross-sections at representative levels is shown.

Section I

The Whole Brain and Features of a Midsagittal Section

The figures in this section show 1. the relationship of the parts of the brain stem to the cerebral hemisphere and 2. the relationships of the cranial nerves to the external features of the ventral aspect of the brain stem.

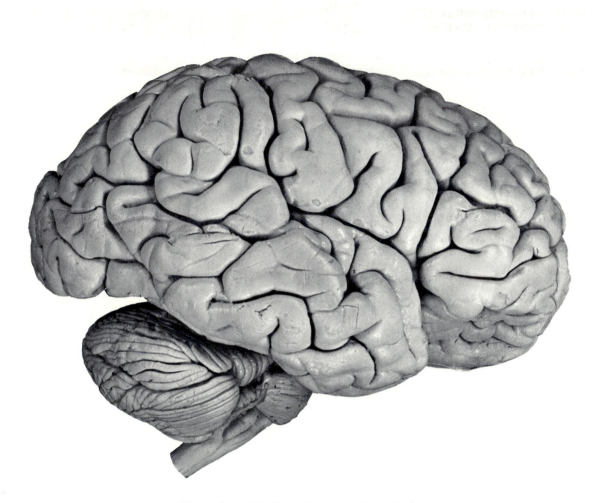

Figure 1a and b. Lateral Aspect of the Brain.

Observations

The brain has a segmented, midline portion called the *brain stem* that is largely concealed by its appendages, the cerebral hemispheres and the cerebellum. The right and left cerebral hemispheres are attached to the sides of the diencephalon. The cerebellum is attached to the dorsal surface of the pons segment.

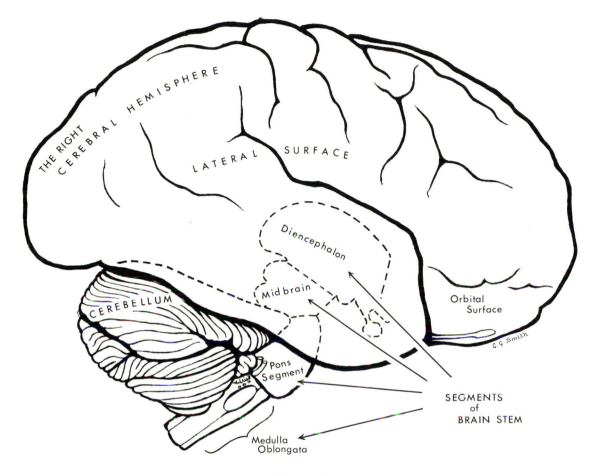

Figure 1b.

The outline of the diencephalon, the midbrain and the upper portion of the pons segment is shown in the accompanying drawing projected onto the lateral aspect of the cerebral hemisphere.

The cerebral hemisphere has lateral, medial, and inferior surfaces. The anterior part of the inferior surface rests on the roof of the orbit and faces laterally as well as inferiorly.

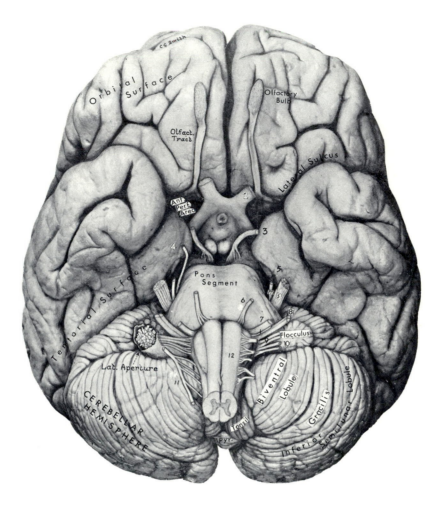

Figure 2a and b. Basal (ventral) Aspect of the Brain.

Observations

1. The olfactory nerve fibers enter the olfactory bulb like the bristles of a brush. They are torn away when the bulb is peeled off the cribriform plate in removing the brain.

2. The optic chiasma is at the rostral end of the brain stem.

3. The third nerve emerges medial to the pathway for voluntary movement located in the crus cerebri. The sixth nerve penetrates this pathway as it emerges from the pons to form the pyramid, and the twelfth nerve emerges at the lateral border of the pyramid. Lesions of these nerves may, therefore, be associated with paralysis of voluntary movement of the arm and leg on the opposite side of the body.

4. The fourth cranial nerve emerges from the back of the brain stem and courses ventrally, lateral to the crus cerebri, to accompany the third nerve into the orbit.

5. The Nervus Intermedius is the sensory root of the facial nerve. It conveys impulses from taste endings on the anterior two-thirds of the tongue.

6. The anterior and posterior perforated areas are the areas where thread-like vessels enter and leave the brain. The

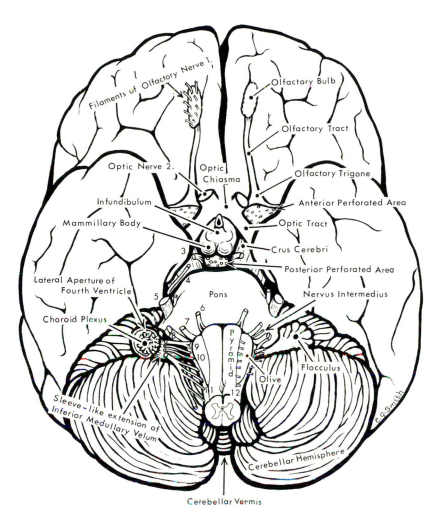

Figure 2b.

anterior perforated area is on the ventral surface of the hemisphere immediately lateral to the optic chiasma and tract. Vessels entering the hemisphere here supply the pathway for voluntary movement. Occlusion of these vessels results in paralysis of the opposite side of the body. The posterior perforated area is coextensive with the ventral surface of the midbrain and is located between the right and left crura cerebri.

7. The lateral aperture is an opening at the lateral angle of the inferior velum, that is, the membranous roof of the fourth ventricle. Through this perforation cerebrospinal fluid formed in the ventricles

escapes into the subarachnoid space. It is usually at the end of a short sleeve-like extension of the inferior velum that extends laterally between the flocculus and the rootlets of nerves 9 and 10. On the right side (left side of Figure 2) the sleeve-like tube is abnormally long. On the left side the tubular extension is short and hidden by the rootlets of the ninth and tenth nerves.

8. The cerebellum is shaped like a dumbbell. Its median constricted part is called the vermis portion; its large lateral portions are the cerebellar hemispheres.

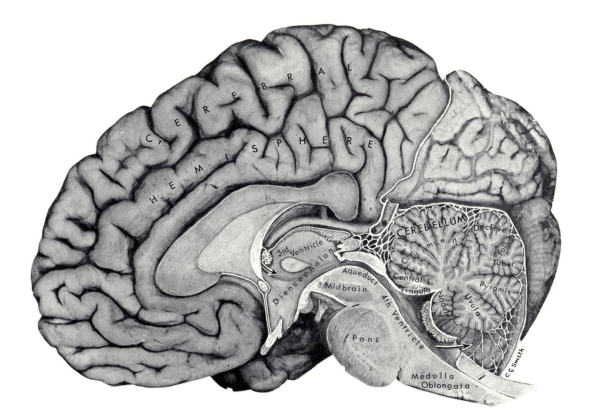

Figure 3a and b. Midsagittal Section of the Brain.

Observations

1. The arachnoid membrane is a translucent membrane that encloses the brain without entering the sulci of the cerebral hemispheres or the cerebellum. In this preparation the arachnoid was removed except where it covered the cerebellum and the occipital lobe of the cerebral hemisphere. The arachnoid membrane forms the wall of an enlargement of the subarachnoid space called the cerebellomedullary cistern. Cerebrospinal fluid may be drained from this cistern by inserting a needle in the suboccipital region.

2. The superior medullary velum of the fourth ventricle contains the lingula, a thin lobule of the cerebellum labeled on the photograph. The inferior velum contains a choroid plexus and has three apertures, two lateral (see Figure 2) and

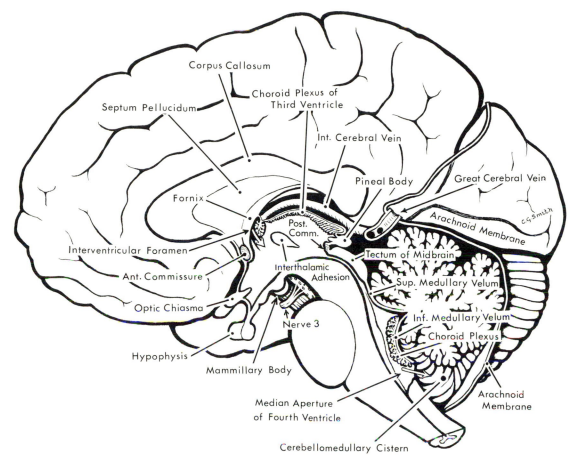

Corpus Callosum
Choroid Plexus of
Third Ventricle
Septum Pellucidum
Int. Cerebral Vein
Pineal Body
Great Cerebral Vein
Fornix
Arachnoid Membrane
Post.
Comm.
Interventricular Foramen
Tectum of Midbrain
Interthalamic
Adhesion
Ant. Commissure
Sup. Medullary Velum
Optic Chiasma
Inf. Medullary Velum
Nerve 3
Choroid Plexus
Hypophysis
Mammillary Body
Arachnoid
Membrane
Median Aperture
of Fourth Ventricle
Cerebellomedullary Cistern

Figure 3b.

one median. Occlusion of these apertures blocks escape of cerebrospinal fluid from the ventricles and is one cause of hydrocephalus.

3. The interventricular foramen is located at the anterior superior angle of the third ventricle. The choroid plexus of the lateral ventricle extends medially in the roof of this foramen.

4. The anterior commissure connects the cerebral cortex of the right and the left temporal lobes. The posterior commissure is a part of the light reflex pathway. Light entering one eye excites constriction of the pupils of both eyes.

5. The interthalamic adhesion is an adhesion uniting the walls of the third ventricle. It varies in size and was absent in 14 of 52 brains examined by the author.

Section II

Serial Dissections of the Lateral Aspect of the Cerebral Hemisphere

Progressive dissection of the lateral aspect of the hemisphere uncovers in turn 1) the association bundle connecting cortical areas essential to comprehension; 2) the association bundle relating areas essential to problem solving; 3) the fan-shaped layer of fibers (projection fibers) that connect all cortical areas with the brain stem (The marginal part of this fan is called the corona radiata; the handle of the fan is called the internal capsule. The internal capsule forms the medial part of the capsule of the lentiform nucleus, a relay station that shows degenerative changes in paralysis agitans. Hemorrhage into the internal capsule is one cause of stroke.); and 4) the parts of the lateral ventricle. The extent of the cavity can be palpated and then opened by removing fibers of the corona radiata. In doing so, the structures in the medial wall of the ventricle are exposed.

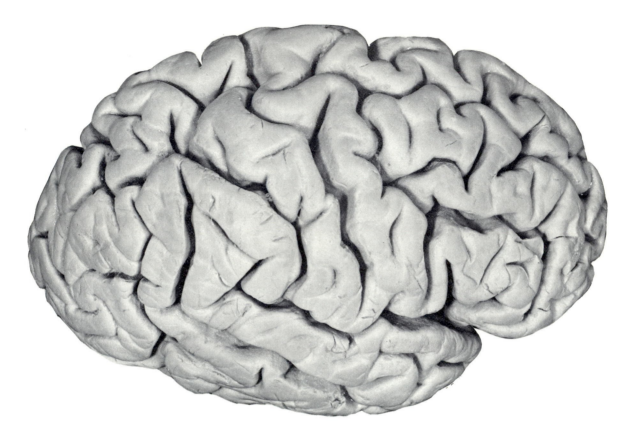

Figure 4a and b. Lateral Aspect of the Right Cerebral Hemisphere.

Observations

1. Each gyrus of the cerebral hemisphere is a fold of cerebral cortex (a thin layer of gray matter) with a core of white matter. The furrows are called sulci. The pattern of sulci and gyri attained shortly before birth is recognizable in some adult brains, as shown in this specimen. Usually the expanding cortex acquires secondary foldings that make identification of this basic pattern difficult.

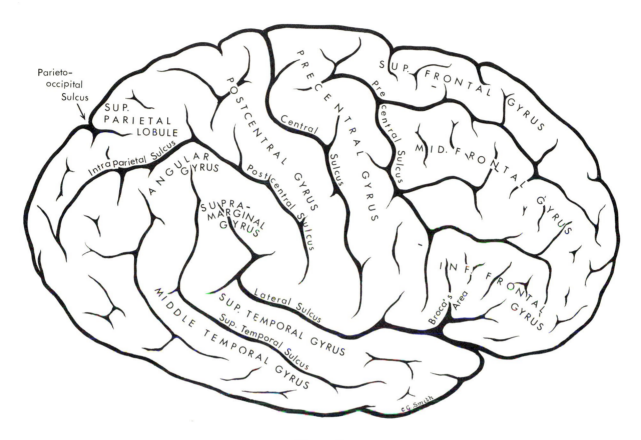

Figure 4b.

2. The lateral sulcus has an extensive floor called the insula.

3. The central sulcus separates the general sensory area in the postcentral gyrus from the motor area in the precentral gyrus.

4. The angular gyrus, the supramarginal gyrus, and the posterior part of the inferior frontal gyrus (Broca's Area) are association areas that in the dominant hemisphere, usually the left, are part of the speech mechanism.

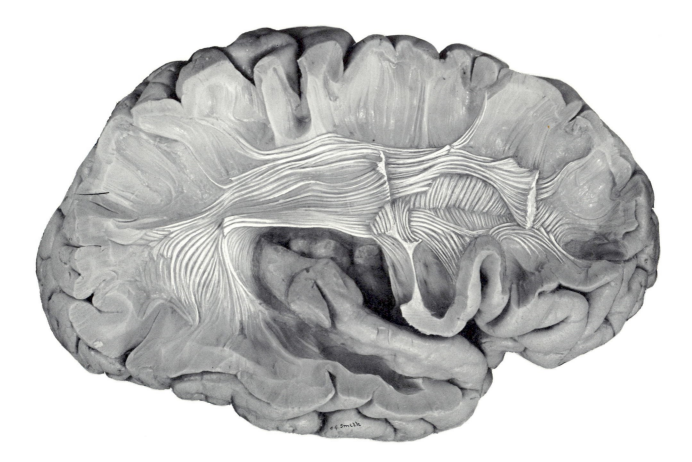

Figure 5a and b. The First Stage in Dissection of the Cerebral Hemisphere (lateral approach).

Dissection

To dissect the cerebral hemisphere using the lateral approach, the cortex and short association fibers around the lateral sulcus are removed.

Observations

1. The superior longitudinal fasciculus is a bundle of long association fibers. An important function of these fibers is to convey impulses to the association cortex of the parietal lobe.

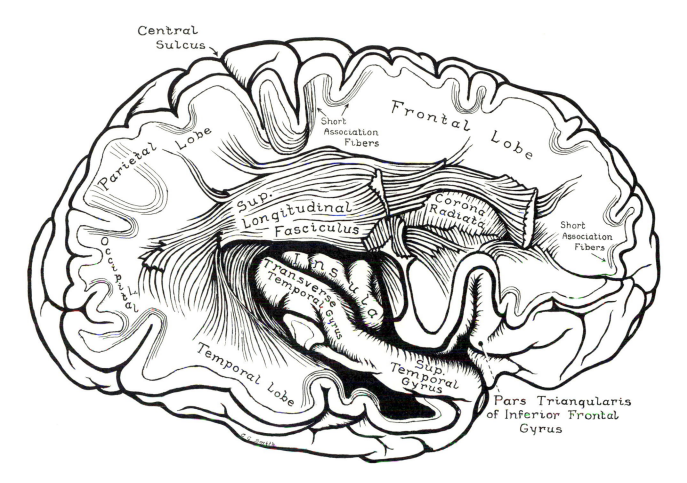

Figure 5b.

Clinical Note

2. The cortex of the transverse temporal gyrus is the auditory sensory area. It is located on the lower wall of the lateral sulcus.

A lesion of the superior longitudinal fasciculus will greatly impair the function of the parietal association area (ability to identify objects) because the input from the sensory areas will be cut off. If the lesion is in the dominant hemisphere, the ability to understand written or spoken words will be lost.

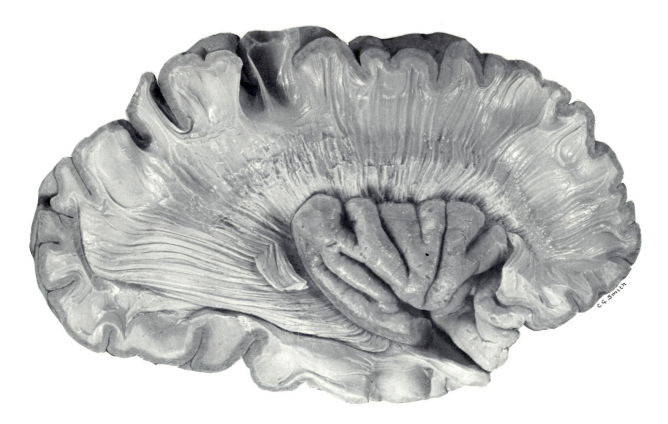

Figure 6a and b. The Second Stage in Dissection of the Cerebral Hemisphere (lateral approach).

Dissection	*Observations*
Removal of the superior longitudinal fasciculus.	1. The insula is an island of cortex that forms the floor of the lateral sulcus. Its inferior angle is called the limen.
	2. The corona radiata is a crown-like ridge along the superior border of the insula

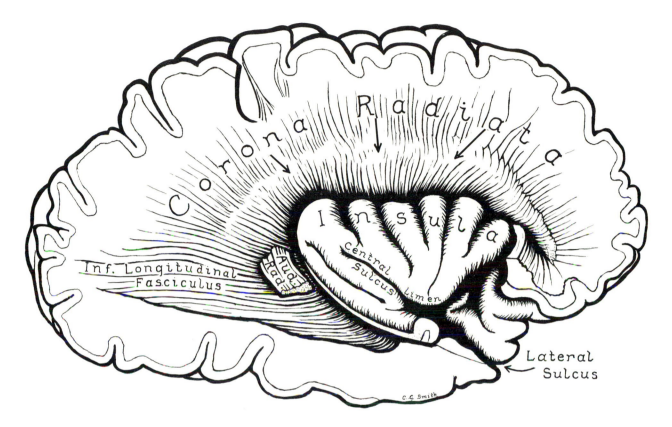

Figure 6b.

where fibers connecting the cortex with lower levels of the brain intersect commissural fibers connecting the two hemispheres.

3. The inferior longitudinal fasciculus is a bundle of long association fibers. It extends anteriorly deep to the inferior portion of the insula.

4. The fibers of the auditory pathway, called the auditory radiation, have been cut where they enter the core of the transverse temporal gyrus.

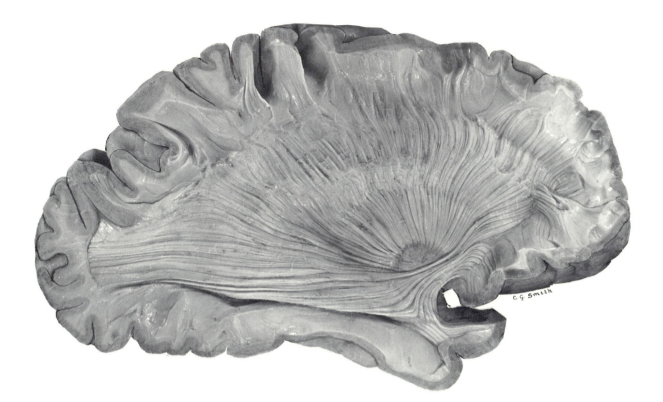

Figure 7a and b. The Third Stage in Dissection of the Cerebral Hemisphere (lateral approach).

Dissection

Removal of the cortex of the insula and its underlying short association fibers.

Observations

1. The inferior longitudinal fasciculus and the uncinate fasciculus convey data from recognition areas of cortex (parietal, occipital, and temporal) and from cortex that functions as a memory bank (temporal) to the highest levels of association in the frontal lobe.

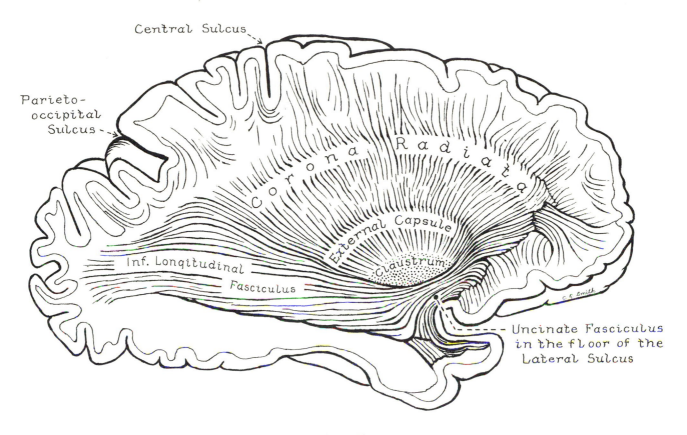

Figure 7b.

2. The external capsule is comprised of a thin layer of fibers that passes between two of the central nuclei of the cerebral hemisphere; namely, the claustrum that is superficial to it, and the lentiform nucleus that is deep to it.

Clinical Note

Lesions of the frontal association cortex impair ability to solve problems. A similar loss of function may occur in lesions of the inferior longitudinal and uncinate fasciculi.

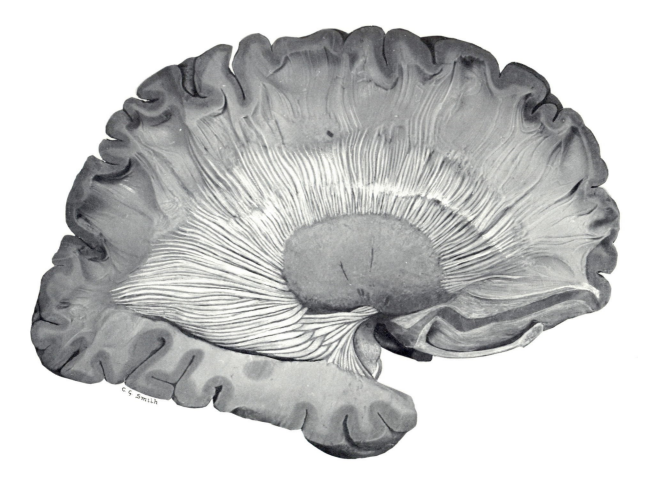

Figure 8a and b. The Fourth Stage in Dissection of the Cerebral Hemisphere (lateral approach).

Dissection

Removal of the inferior longitudinal and uncinate fasciculi, the claustrum, and the external capsule.

Observations

1. The lentiform nucleus extends to the inferior surface of the hemisphere where it is called the anterior perforated substance.
2. The fibers of the optic radiation convey impulses from the right half of the retina of each eye. As these fibers emerge from deep to the lentiform nucleus, they fan out coursing first toward the temporal pole, then toward the occipital pole. The

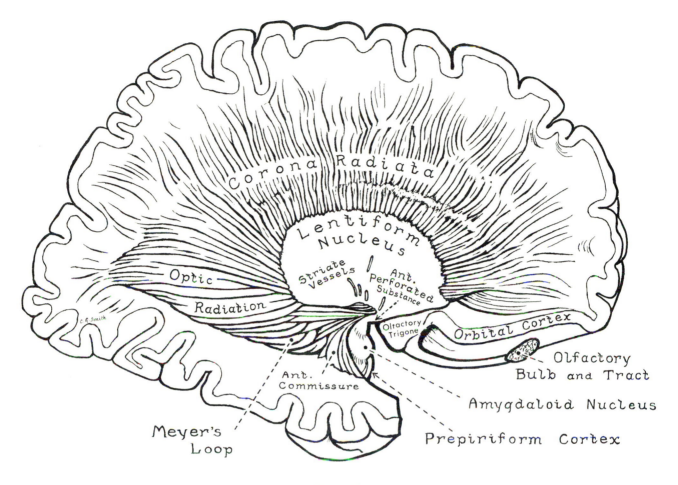

Figure 8b.

fibers extending closest to the temporal pole convey impulses from the lower portion of each retina and are known as Meyer's Loop.
3. The anterior commissure connects areas of cortex of the right and left temporal lobes. These areas serve, in part, as a memory bank.
4. The amygdaloid nucleus forms part of the medial surface of the temporal pole.
5. The olfactory trigone is a terminus for some of the fibers of the olfactory tract.

Clinical Notes

1. The striate vessels penetrating the anterior perforated substance supply the pyramidal tract located in the internal capsule. Occlusion or rupture of these vessels is one cause of stroke.
2. Injuries of the temporal pole may involve the fibers of Meyer's Loop. Interruption of these fibers will result in blindness in the lower right quadrant of the retina of both eyes.

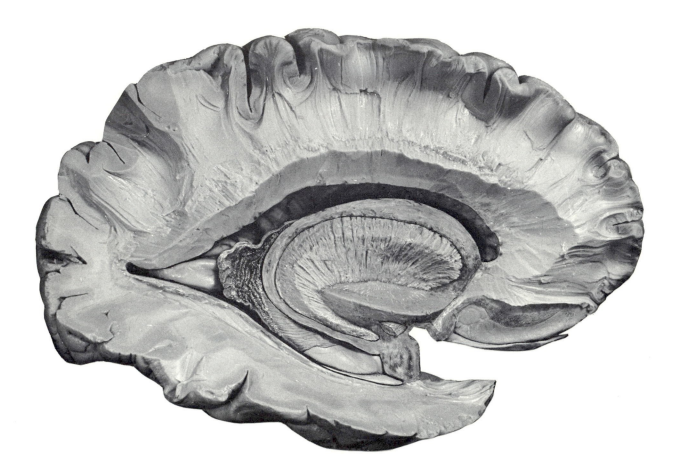

Figure 9a and b. The Fifth Stage in Dissection of the Cerebral Hemisphere (lateral approach).

Dissection

Removal of the wall of the lateral ventricle, the marginal part of the internal capsule, the lateral portion of the anterior commissure, and the upper half of the lentiform nucleus.

Observations

1. The internal capsule is a fan-shaped band of fibers that forms part of a cone.

Lodged within the cone is the lentiform nucleus. Anteriorly, where the cone is incomplete, the lentiform nucleus is connected with the large anterior end of the caudate nucleus. The caudate nucleus, as its name implies, is a tapered, tail-like mass of gray matter. It extends back, medial to the fibers of the internal capsule where it forms in turn a part of the wall of the anterior horn, the body, and the inferior horn of the lateral ventricle. At the tip of the inferior horn the attenu-

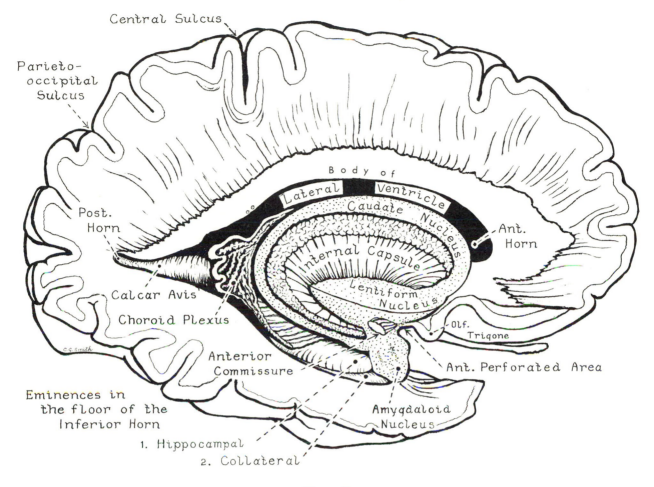

Figure 9b.

ated caudate nucleus is connected with the amygdaloid nucleus.

2. The calcar avis is an elevation in the wall of the posterior horn of the lateral ventricle. It is produced by the deep calcarine sulcus on the medial surface of the occipital lobe. The hippocampal and collateral eminences are similarly produced by deep sulci on the medial aspect of the temporal lobe, that is by the hippocampal and collateral sulci, respectively.

Clinical Notes

The enlargement of the choroid plexus anterior to the posterior horn commonly contains cysts, caseous masses, and calcified nodules. Calcified nodules, if present, can serve as points of reference for the radiologist.

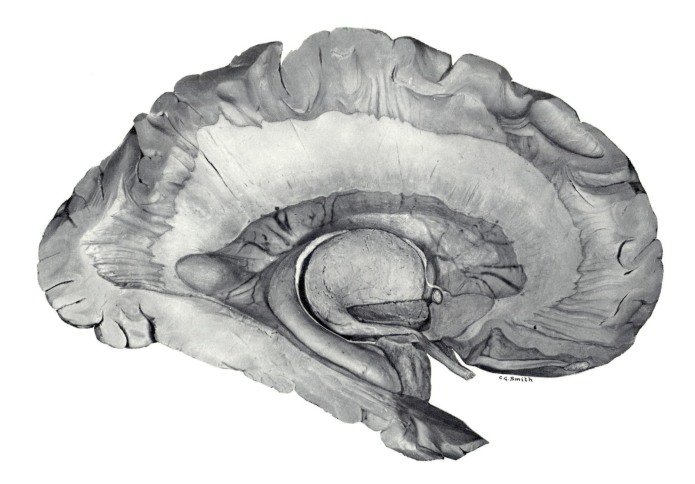

Figure 10a and b. The Sixth Stage in Dissection of the Cerebral Hemisphere (lateral approach).

Dissection

Removal of the lower half of the lentiform nucleus, the internal capsule, the caudate nucleus, and the choroid plexus of the lateral ventricle.

Observations

1. The septum pellucidum is a translucent membrane that separates the right and left lateral ventricles.

2. The fornix is the efferent fiber bundle of the cortex of the hippocampal formation. This cortex forms the wall of the deep hippocampal sulcus (*see* Figure 11) that is responsible for the hippocampal eminence. Fibers of this cortex form a thin layer on the ventricular aspect of the eminence and then course along its medial border to reach the midline. There they turn anteriorly along the lower border of the septum pellucidum to enter the diencephalon just in front of the interventricular foramen.

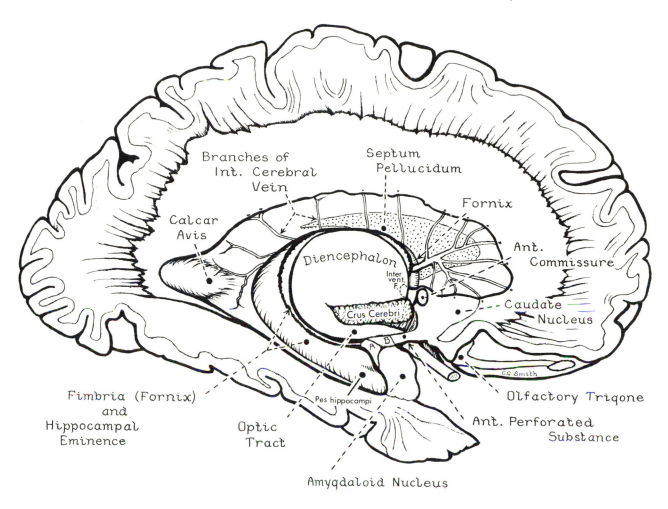

Figure 10b.

3. The area on the amygdaloid nucleus labeled "A" is the extent of its attachment to the tail of the caudate nucleus. The area labeled "B" is the extent of its attachment to the lentiform nucleus.

Clinical Note

A hole may be present in the septum pellucidum, providing an abnormal communication between the two lateral ventricles. A perforation was found in four of 52 brains examined by the author.

If the septum pellucidum is not perforated, air introduced into the lateral ventricle can only reach the third ventricle by way of the interventricular foramen. If the septum is perforated, it may reach the third ventricle through the interventricular foramen of the opposite side.

Section III

Serial Dissections of the Medial Aspect of the Cerebral Hemisphere

Progressive dissection of the medial aspect of the hemisphere reveals in turn 1. the association bundle (cingulum) that connects cortical areas of the lateral aspect of the hemisphere with the cortex of the cingulate gyrus (data integrated in the cingulate gyrus give rise to emotional feelings); 2. the radiating fibers of the corpus callosum that connect cortical areas of the right and left hemispheres; 3. the pathway descending from the cingulate gyrus to the brain stem, to excite emotional responses (the dentate gyrus and the hippocampus are relay stations of this pathway and the fornix is the terminal part); and 4. the parts of the lateral ventricle.

The extent of this cavity can be appreciated by palpation and its medial wall can be removed by cutting across the fibers of the corpus callosum and the fornix. In doing so, the structures in the lateral wall of the ventricle are revealed. These structures can then be seen without removing the diencephalon. However, in the last of this series of dissections of the medial aspect of the hemisphere, this portion of the brain stem was removed along with the ependymal lining of the ventricle. This was done in order to obtain a photograph of the full extent of the caudate nucleus and the radiating fibers of the corpus callosum in its wall.

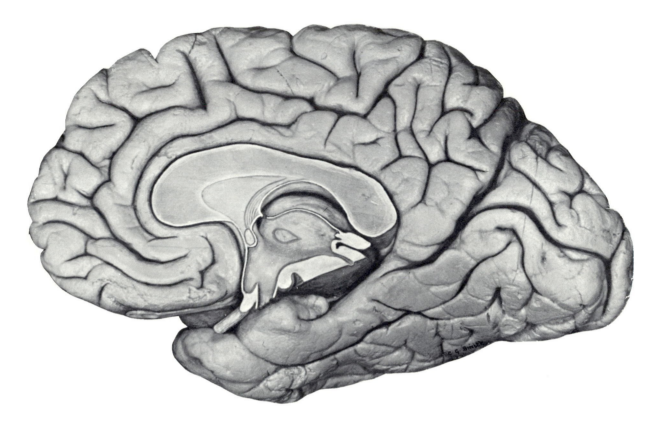

Figure 11a and b. Medial Aspect of the Right Cerebral Hemisphere.

Observations

1. The corpus callosum is comprised of a thick, strap-like band of fibers connecting the two hemispheres. Its thin anterior border is attached to the diencephalon; its thick posterior border is free and is called the splenium.

2. The septum pellucidum is a thin part of the medial wall of the lateral ventricle. There is one for each hemisphere. They are usually closely applied and adhere, except anteriorly. The small anterior space between the two may become distended with fluid and then is known as a cyst of the septum pellucidum.

3. The fornix is comprised of a bundle of fibers in the lower border of the septum pellucidum. It conveys impulses from the cortex in the hippocampal sulcus to the brain stem. It enters the diencephalon just behind the anterior commissure.

4. The anterior commissure is comprised of a bundle of commissural fibers connecting the cortex of the right and left temporal lobes.

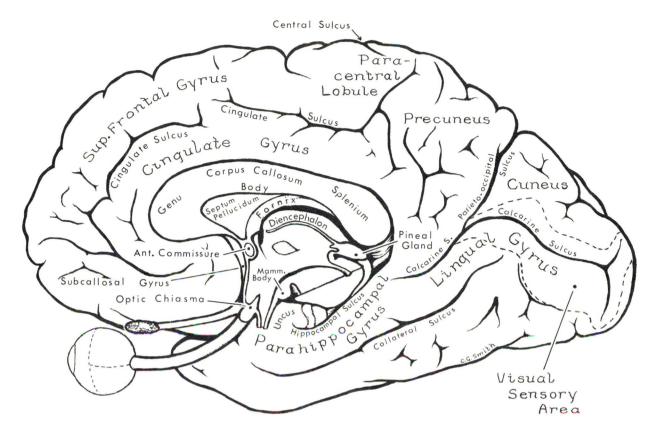

Figure 11b.

5. The cingulate and parahippocampal gyri are connected behind the splenium. This ring-like band of cortex is known as the limbic lobe.

6. The cortex in the walls of the deep calcarine sulcus receives visual impulses. The right hemisphere receives impulses from the right half of each eye. The upper part of the retina projects to the upper wall of the sulcus, the lower part to the lower wall of the sulcus.

7. The parieto-occipital sulcus separates the parietal and occipital lobes.

8. The paracentral lobule unites the precentral and postcentral gyri around the end of the central sulcus, on the medial surface of the hemisphere. The motor area for the foot is in the anterior part of the lobule, the sensory area for the foot is in the posterior part.

9. The hippocampal sulcus is at the medial border of the parahippocampal gyrus. It extends from the splenium to the union of the parahippocampal gyrus and the uncus.

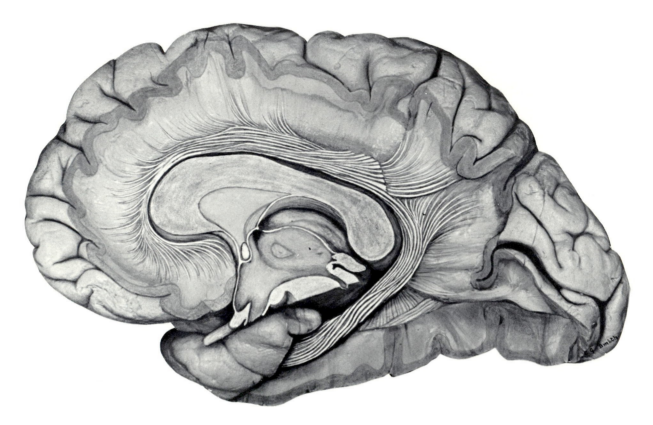

Figure 12a and b. The First Stage in Dissection of the Medial Aspect of the Right Cerebral Hemisphere exposure of the cingulum.

Dissection

The cingulum is comprised of a bundle of long association fibers in the core of the cingulate and parahippocampal gyri. To expose it, the cortex and short association fibers were removed from the medial aspect of the hemisphere. Fibers enter the cingulum from the cortex of the frontal, parietal, occipital, and temporal lobes. In this preparation the very thin layer of fibers that enters the cingulum from the temporal lobe has been removed in order to expose the deeper fibers of the corpus callosum and a small part of the optic radiation.

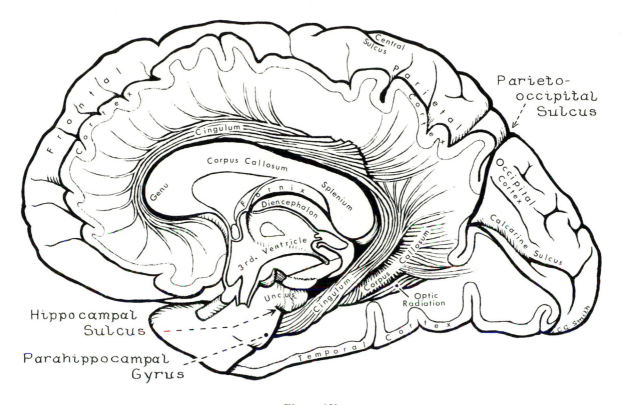

Figure 12b.

Observations

The association fibers of the cingulum convey data to the limbic lobe, i.e. the cingulate and parahippocampal gyri, to excite an awareness of an emotional feeling. To excite an appropriate response, impulses are conveyed by other fibers of the cingulum to the cortex in the wall of the hippocampal sulcus, exposed in figure 13, which gives rise to the fibers of the fornix that arch below the septum pellucidum to enter the diencephalon anterior to the interventricular foramen.

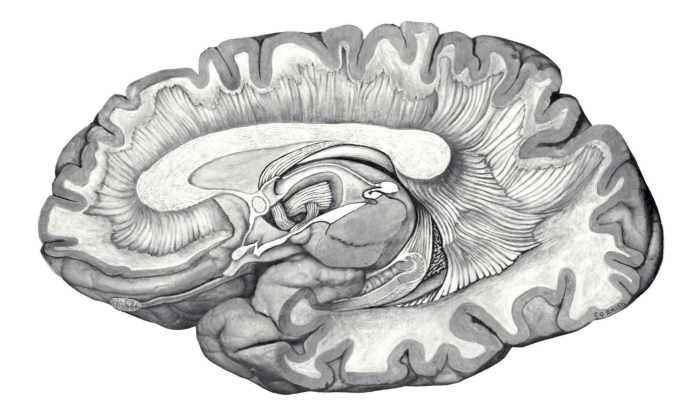

Figure 13a and b. The Second Stage in Dissection of the Medial Aspect of the Right Cerebral Hemisphere.

Dissection

Removal of the cingulum, the cortex in the posterior half of the hippocampal sulcus, and a portion of the wall of the third ventricle to uncover the fornix and the mammillothalamic tract.

Observations

1. The forceps minor and forceps major are the anterior and posterior portions of the corpus callosum, respectively.

2. The hippocampal sulcus begins anteriorly in the angle formed by the union of the parahippocampal gyrus and the uncus. It ends below the splenium. It is lined by a band of archicortex (three layers of cells) that is continuous along its one border with the cortex of the parahippocampal gyrus, but its other border is free. This free border curls back into the sulcus to form a nodular ridge called the dentate gyrus. The relationship of the dentate gyrus to the hippocampus can be seen where they are cut across in this dissection.

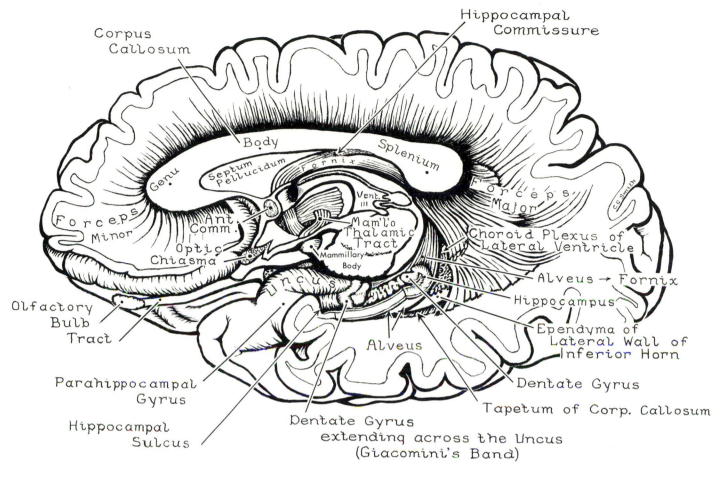

Figure 13b.

3. The alveus is a thin layer of fibers that covers the ventricular aspect of the cortex in the hippocampal sulcus. The fibers of the alveus have their origin in the hippocampal cortex and come together to form the fornix. This bundle extends to the midline where it courses anteriorly to form the inferior border of the septum pellucidum. It leaves the septum pellucidum to enter the diencephalon just in front of the interventricular foramen and behind the anterior commissure. The fibers that reach the diencephalon end in the mammillary body. They are projection fibers. Some fibers of the fornix cross the midline to form the hippocampal commissure which connects the hippocampal cortex of the right and the left hemispheres.

4. The mammillothalamic tract emerges from the medial part of the mammillary body to end in the anterior thalamic nucleus of the diencephalon. It has been traced in this dissection to where it penetrates the fibers connecting the medial nucleus of the thalamus with the frontal lobe cortex.

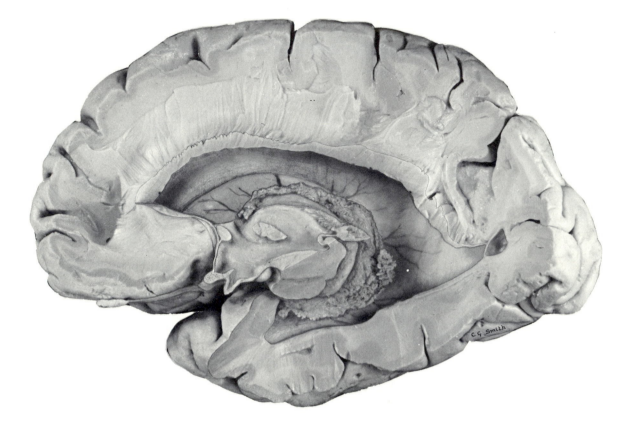

Figure 14a and b. The Third Stage in Dissection of the Medial Aspect of the
Cerebral Hemisphere—Interior of the Lateral Ventricle.

Dissection

1. Insert a probe into the interventricular foramen to the tip of the anterior horn of the lateral ventricle and cut down on it to sever the fornix, the septum pellucidum, and the anterior part of the corpus callosum.

2. Extend the cut in the corpus callosum posteriorly in a parasagittal plane, about 2 cm from the midline as far as the splenium; then, following the outer border of the ventricle, cut to the tip of the posterior horn and continue on as far as the tip of the inferior horn.

3. Break the delicate membrane connecting the choroid plexus to the border of the fornix.

4. Complete the detachment of the "medial" wall of the lateral ventricle by cutting across the uncus and the amygdaloid nucleus.

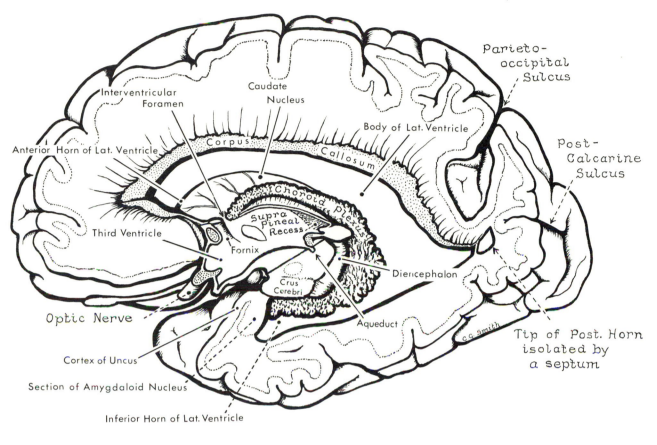

Figure 14b.

Observations

1. The "lateral" wall of the lateral ventricle is formed by the caudate and the amygdaloid nuclei and by white matter (*see* Figure 15). A thin layer of epithelial cells, the ependyma, forms the lining of the ventricle.

2. The choroid plexus extends from the interventricular foramen to the tip of the inferior horn. It does not enter the anterior or the posterior horns.

3. The tip of the posterior horn is isolated from the rest of the lateral ventricle by a septum in this specimen. This is an anomaly.

4. The suprapineal recess is an outpouching of the roof of the third ventricle.

5. The vessels deep to the ependyma are tributaries of the internal cerebral vein.

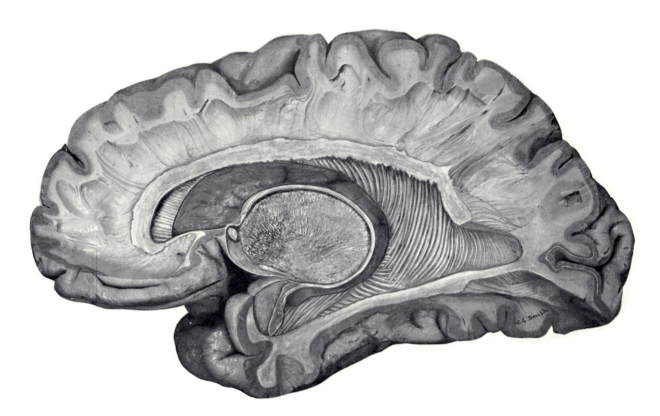

Figure 15a and b. The Fourth Stage in Dissection of the Medial
Aspect of the Cerebral Hemisphere—Structures in the
"Lateral" Wall of the Lateral Ventricle.

Dissection

The diencephalon was detached from the hemisphere and removed along with the choroid plexus of the lateral ventricle. The ependyma was stripped off the lateral wall except where it covered the caudate nucleus and the amygdaloid nucleus.

Observations

1. The caudate nucleus almost completely encircles the area where the cerebral hemisphere is attached to the diencephalon. The expanded anterior end of the caudate nucleus forms the greater part of the wall of the anterior horn, that is, the portion of the ventricle in front of the interventricular foramen. From here the nucleus tapers as far as the tip of the inferior horn where it is attached to the bulb-like amygdaloid nucleus. Note that the amygdaloid nucleus extends anterior to the inferior horn and reaches the external surface to form part of the uncus.

2. The fibers seen anterior to the head of the caudate nucleus are projection fibers that are an extension of those that form the anterior limb of the internal capsule. The commissural fibers of the corpus callosum form almost all the rest of the wall of the ventricle. Those fibers in the wall of the posterior and inferior horns

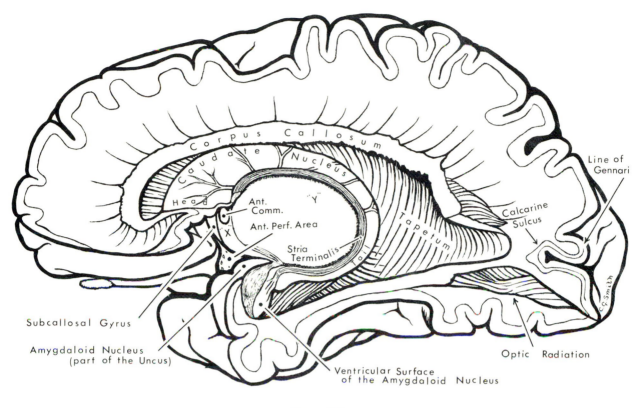

Figure 15b.

form a very thin layer called the tape-tum. At the tip of the inferior horn the wall is formed by projection fibers of the sublenticular limb of the internal capsule.

3. The fibers that were cut to detach the diencephalon are fibers of the internal capsule, area "Y."

4. Immediately anterior to the anterior commissure the thickness of the wall of the lateral ventricle is formed by gray matter of the subcallosal gyrus, a portion of the septal area of the medial wall of the ventricle.

5. The stria terminalis conveys impulses from the amygdaloid nucleus to the hy-pothalamus of the diencephalon. It courses deep to the ependyma, along the inner border of the caudate nucleus, to enter the diencephalon just behind the anterior commissure.

6. Area "X" just below the anterior commissure is gray matter connecting the septal region of the hemisphere with the hypothalamus of the diencephalon.

7. The line of Gennari is a thin layer of myelinated fibers in the cortex of the calcarine sulcus. It is formed by the terminals of the fibers of the optic radiation which end in the fourth cortical layer, thus dividing it into superficial and deep portions.

Section IV

External Features of the Brain Stem

The brain stem is the midline portion of the brain. It is the definitive cephalic part of the embryonic neural tube. It has three primary subdivisions: forebrain, midbrain, and hindbrain. Of these, the forebrain is divided into a rostral part, the telencephalon, and a caudal part, the diencephalon.

The greater part of the telencephalon is evaginated early in the course of development to form the cerebral hemisphere. Therefore, it is acceptable, for practical purposes, to use the term diencephalon for the whole forebrain segment of the brain stem.

The hindbrain is also divided into rostral and caudal parts, the pons segment and the medulla oblongata, respectively. The pons segment has the cerebellum attached to its dorsal surface and is so named because it is covered ventrally by a band of fibers called the pons. These fibers are a part of the major pathway from the cerebral cortex to the cerebellum. They form the middle cerebellar peduncle, also known as the brachium pontis.

The specimen used for Figures 17, 18, and 19 was prepared by 1. detaching the whole of the hemisphere from the right side of the diencephalon and retaining the fibers of the internal capsule and the related lentiform and caudate nuclei on the left side; 2. isolating the three fiber bundles (peduncles) that connect the cerebellum and the brain stem and cutting them to detach the cerebellum; and 3. peeling away the thin, rubbery membrane of neuroglia that partially obscures the fibers of the spinal tract of the fifth nerve and the medial and lateral lemnisci.

The specimen illustrated in Figure 16 was prepared to show the relationships of the diencephalon to the internal capsule and the associated caudate and lentiform nuclei. For this purpose the dorsal portion of the diencephalon, the caudate, and the lentiform nuclei were sliced off, leaving the fibers of the internal capsule in place. Compare this dissection with the horizontal section of the hemisphere shown in Figure 29.

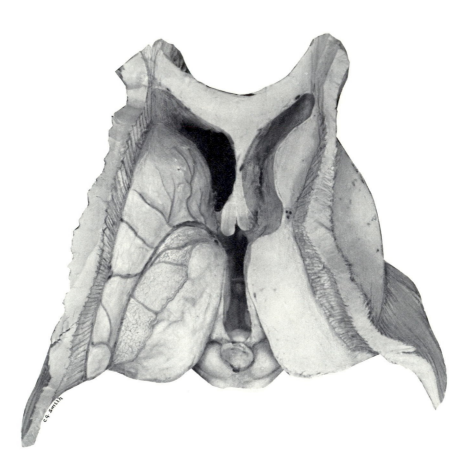

Figure 16a and b. Dorsal Aspect of the Diencephalon Showing its Relationships.

Dissection

The dorsal surface of the diencephalon has been exposed by dissecting away all portions of the two hemispheres except the inferior part of the septum pellucidum, the anterior portion of the corpus callosum, the internal capsule, the caudate nucleus, and the lentiform nucleus.

On the right side the diencephalon, the caudate and lentiform nuclei have been cut horizontally at the level of the interventricular foramen. The fibers of the internal capsule have also been cut horizontally but at a slightly higher level.

Observations

1. The anterior angle of the dorsal (superior) surface of the diencephalon is penetrated by the right and left fornix.
2. The posterior commissure, which contains the pupillary light-reflex pathways, can be seen because the membranous roof of the third ventricle has been removed.

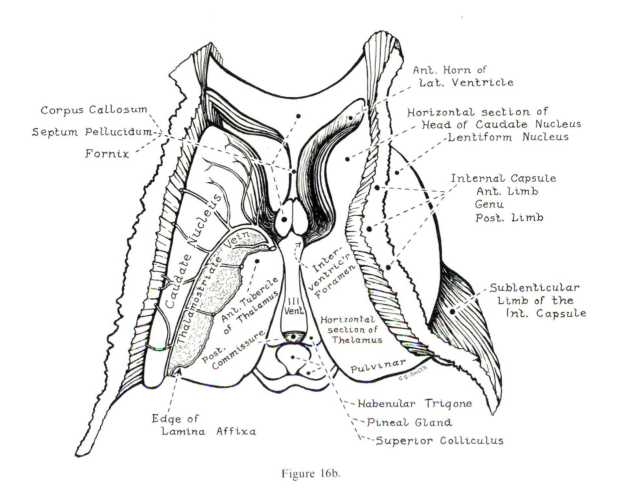

Figure 16b.

3. The anterior tubercle is a nucleus of the thalamus, a dorsal portion of the diencephalon. The interventricular foramen is between the anterior tubercle and the fornix.

4. The pulvinar is that portion of the diencephalon that projects posteriorly above and to the side of the superior colliculus, a portion of the midbrain.

5. The habenular trigone is a portion of the diencephalon called the epithalamus.

6. The walls of the anterior horn of the lateral ventricle are 1) the head of the caudate nucleus, 2) the corpus callosum, and 3) the septum pellucidum.

7. The lamina affixa is a portion of the choroid membrane of the medial wall of the lateral ventricle, that is adhering to the dorsal surface of the diencephalon.

8. The four named portions of the internal capsule are labeled. The anterior limb is between the head of the caudate nucleus and the lentiform nucleus. The posterior and sublenticular limbs separate the lentiform nucleus from the diencephalon and the caudate nucleus.

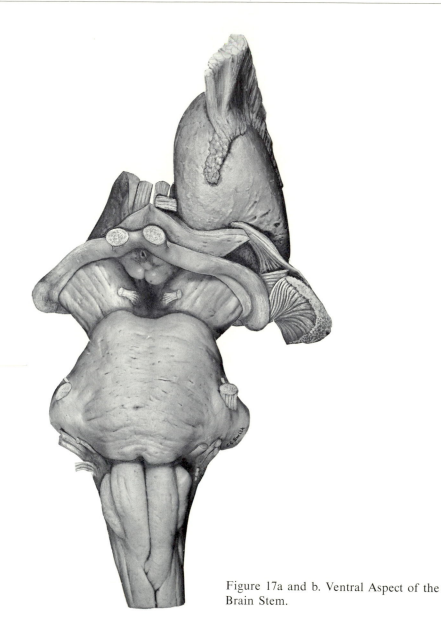

Figure 17a and b. Ventral Aspect of the Brain Stem.

Dissection

The brain stem has been exposed by removing the cerebellum, all of the right cerebral hemisphere, and the major portion of the left hemisphere.

Observations

1. The brain stem has four segments called the medulla oblongata, the pons, the midbrain, and the diencephalon. The features of the ventral surface of the medulla are the pyramids. The pons segment is identified by the transverse fiber band called the pons. The features of the midbrain are the right and the left crus cerebri and the posterior perforated area located between them in the interpeduncular fossa (not labeled). The ventral surface of the diencephalon is small; its features are the lamina terminalis, the optic nerves, the chiasma, the optic tract,

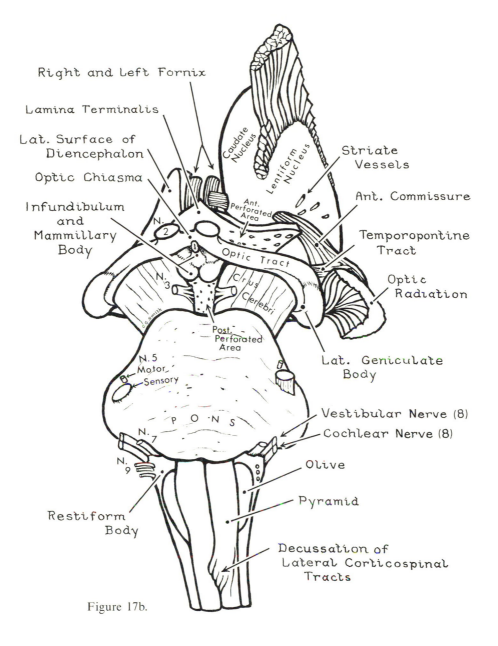

Figure 17b.

the lateral geniculate body, the mammillary bodies, and the infundibulum.

2. The lamina terminalis is the anterior end of the brain stem and forms the thin anterior wall of the third ventricle, the cavity of the diencephalon.

3. The lateral geniculate body has an elevated lateral part and a depressed medial part known as the hilum. It is a cell mass that relays impulses from the optic tract fibers, along the fibers of the optic radiation, to the the visual cortex.

4. The fifth cranial nerve has a sensory and a motor root. It differs from a spinal nerve in that its sensory root is much larger than its motor root and enters the brain *ventral* to the motor root.

5. The decussation of the fibers of the pyramid, forming the lateral corticospinal tract, can be seen clearly in this specimen because the fibers are crossing superficially and in large bundles.

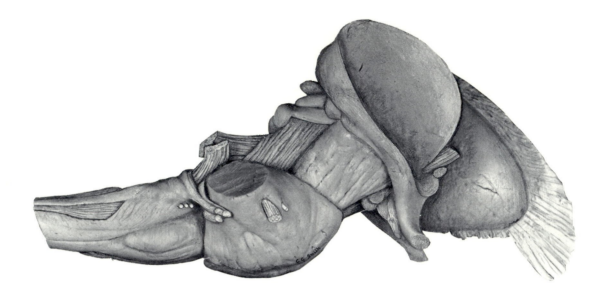

Figure 18a and b. Lateral Aspect of the Brain Stem.

Dissection

Prepared as in Figure 17.

Observations

1. The eighth (vestibulocochlear) nerve has two portions. The vestibular portion is a special position-sense nerve. The cochlear portion mediates the special sense of hearing. These two nerves utilize the same connective tissue sheath until they reach the brain stem. There the major portion of the cochlear division passes dorsal to the restiform body while the vestibular portion passes ventral to it.

2. The spinal tract of the fifth cranial nerve contains the pain and temperature fibers of the trigeminal nerve. It comes to the surface of the medulla to form the external feature called the tuberculum cinereum. It has been defined in this preparation by removing a thin layer of

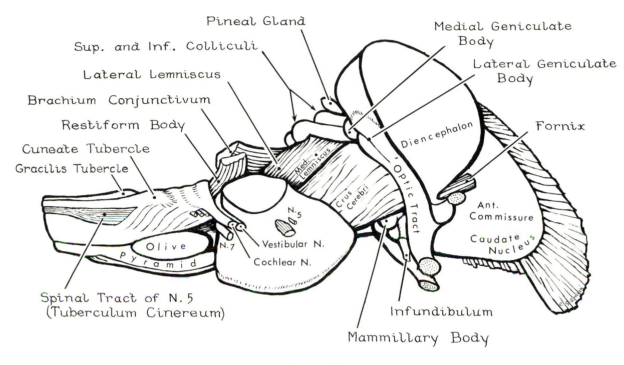

Figure 18b.

supporting tissue called the external limiting membrane.

3. There are three bundles of fibers in each half of the stalk of the cerebellum. These were isolated and cut when the cerebellum was removed. The restiform body provides input from all the sense organs. The brachium pontis, labeled in figure 19b, provides input from the cerebral cortex, and the brachium conjunctivum is its efferent bundle.

4. The medial and lateral lemnisci, like the spinal tract of nerve five, have been defined by removing a thin outer covering of supporting tissue. The two lemnisci have come together to form a single ribbon on the lateral aspect of the midbrain. The lateral lemniscus is part of the auditory pathway and the medial lemniscus is made up of two pathways, one for touch and one for position.

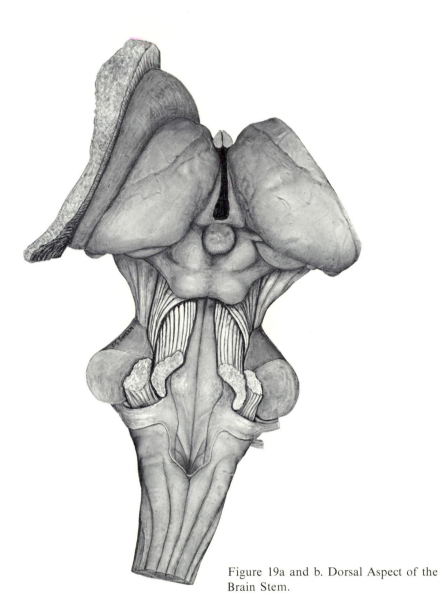

Figure 19a and b. Dorsal Aspect of the Brain Stem.

Dissection

Prepared as in Figure 17.

Observations

1. The ridges formed by the fasciculi gracilis and cuneatus terminate in relay nuclei that form the enlargements known as the tubercle of the nucleus gracilis and the tubercle of the nucleus cuneatus. The fibers leaving these nuclei form the medial lemniscus which passes ventrally and crosses the midline to as-

cend and emerge on the surface of the upper part of the pons segment.

2. The three portions of the roof of the fourth ventricle, the superior velum, the cerebellum, and the inferior velum, shown in Figure 3, have been removed to expose the diamond-shaped floor of this cavity. The floor is formed by gray matter and contains nuclei of the cranial nerves. The sulcus limitans intervenes between the sensory nuclei in the lateral part of the floor, namely, the vestibular and cochlear nuclei, and the motor nuclei in the medial part. The hypoglossal

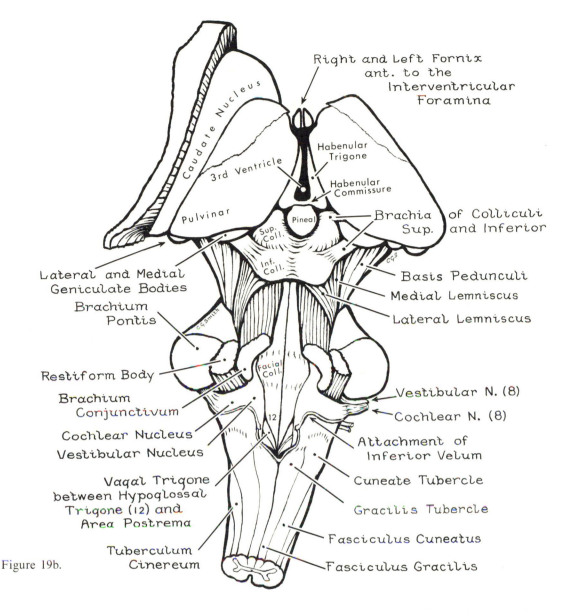

Right and Left Fornix
ant. to the
Interventricular
Foramina

Caudate Nucleus

Habenular
Trigone

3rd Ventricle

Habenular
Commissure

Pulvinar

Pineal

Brachia } of Colliculi
Sup. } and Inferior

Sup. Coll.

Inf. Coll.

Basis Pedunculi

Medial Lemniscus

Lateral Lemniscus

Lateral and Medial
Geniculate Bodies

Brachium
Pontis

C.G.Smith

Facial Coll.

Restiform Body

Vestibular N. (8)

Cochlear N. (8)

Brachium
Conjunctivum

12

Attachment of
Inferior Velum

Cochlear Nucleus
Vestibular Nucleus

Cuneate Tubercle

Vagal Trigone
between Hypoglossal
Trigone (12) and
Area Postrema

Gracilis Tubercle

Fasciculus Cuneatus

Tuberculum
Cinereum

Fasciculus Gracilis

Figure 19b.

trigone contains the motor nucleus of the twelfth nerve, the vagal trigone contains the visceral motor nucleus of the tenth nerve, and the facial colliculus contains the motor nucleus of the sixth cranial nerve. The facial colliculus gets its name because fibers of the facial nerve help to produce the elevation.

3. The area postrema is a specialized cell mass that integrates the vomiting reflex.

4. The right and left superior and inferior colliculi form the dorsal surface of the midbrain and are known as the corpora quadrigemina. The superior colliculi integrate optic reflexes; the inferior colliculi integrate auditory reflexes.

5. The right and the left pulvinar are portions of the base of the wedge-shaped diencephalon that project posteriorly to partially overhang the midbrain.

6. The right and left habenular trigones contain nuclei that are connected by the fibers of the habenular commissure. The midline pineal gland is attached to this commissure.

Section V

Serial Dissections of the Cerebellum

The cerebellum is connected to the back of the pons segment by three bundles called the superior, middle, and inferior cerebellar peduncles. It coordinates the muscles of the body. To do this it receives information from all the sense organs via its inferior peduncle, and information from the cerebral cortex, chiefly via the middle peduncle, but also via the inferior peduncle.

The cerebellum, like the cerebral hemisphere, has an outer covering of gray matter and a core of white matter. Embedded in the core is the dentate nucleus which relays impulses from the cortex to the brain stem and thence by devious pathways to the muscles.

In Figure 20 the main subdivisions of the cerebellar hemisphere are identified. The subdivisions of the vermis, the median part of the dumbbell-shaped cerebellum, are shown in Figure 3. The lobules, anterior to the primary fissure, are parts of the anterior lobe. The rest of the lobules, except for the flocculus, belong to the posterior lobe. The flocculus and the nodule in the vermis belong to a small flocculo-nodular lobe.

The cerebellum is dissected in three stages; 1) the fibers of the middle peduncle are traced into the cerebellum where they form the outer layer of the core of white matter; 2) the fibers of the inferior peduncle are traced into the cerebellum; and 3) are removed to expose the dentate nucleus and the superior peduncle emerging from it.

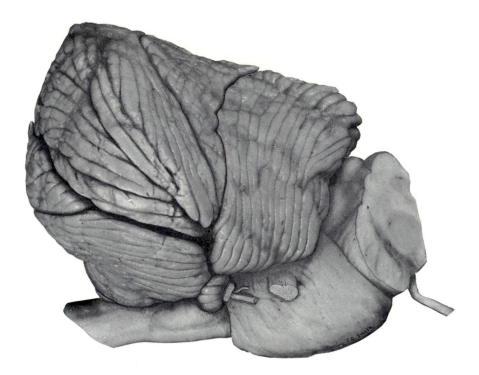

Figure 20a and b. Lateral Aspect of the Cerebellum.

Dissection

The brain stem was sectioned at the level of the midbrain and the upper part of the brain was removed.

Observations

1. The dumbbell-shaped cerebellum (see Figure 2) is divided into lobes and each lobe is divided into lobules by fissures that extend in a lateromedial direction. The lobules of the midline vermis por-

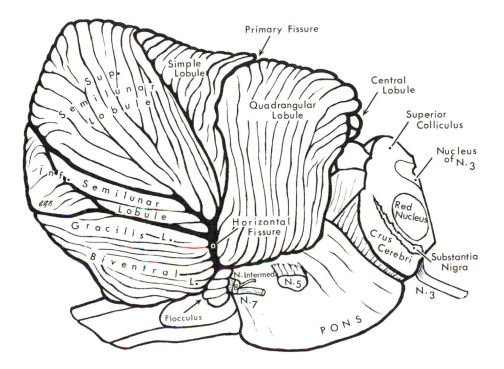

Figure 20b.

tion are labeled in Figures 2 and 3, and the lobules of the hemisphere are labeled in Figures 2 and 20. The nodule of the vermis and the flocculus of the hemisphere make up the flocculonodular lobe, phylogenetically the oldest part of the cerebellum. The rest of the cerebellum is divided into anterior and posterior lobes by the primary fissure.

2. The horizontal fissure separates the superior semilunar and inferior semilunar lobules. In this specimen a deep fissure cuts across the inferior semilunar lobule to complicate the pattern.

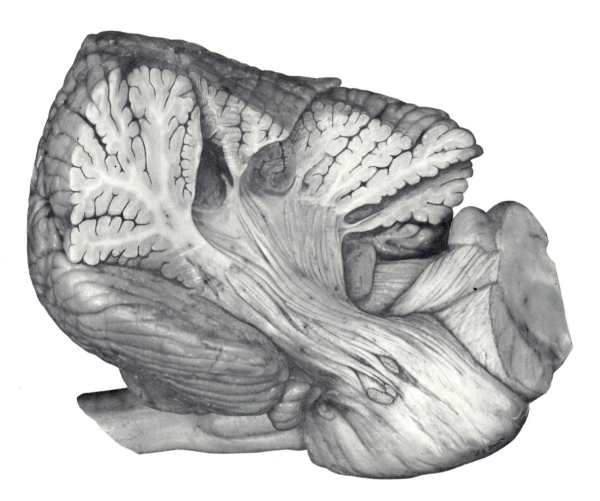

Figure 21a and b. Dissection of the Lateral Aspect of the Cerebellum Exposing the Radiation
of the Middle Cerebellar Peduncle.

Dissection

The fibers of the middle cerebellar peduncle were exposed within the cerebellum by
peeling away the lateral portions of the lobules of the superior surface and the lateral
portion of the inferior semilunar lobule.
The roots of the fifth cranial nerve were

exposed by removing the thin layer of neuroglia that forms the external limiting
membrane of the pons.

Observations

1. Each lobule is attached to the core of
white matter by a band of nerve fibers.
The fibers of the middle cerebellar pe-

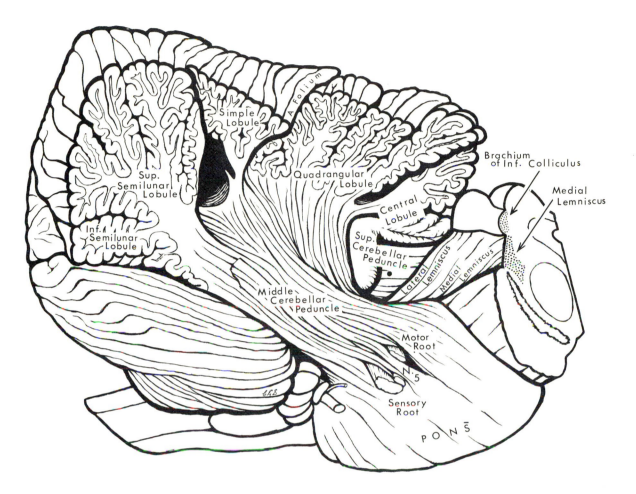

Figure 21b.

duncle form the outer layer of the core and can be seen to extend into each lobule.

2. The motor and sensory roots of the fifth cranial nerve emerge separately. The smaller motor root is dorsal.

3. The fibers of a portion of the superior cerebellar peduncle, as well as the lateral and medial lemniscus, are revealed by removing the external limiting membrane on each of them.

4. The lateral lemniscus and the brachium of the inferior colliculus are parts of the auditory pathway.

5. The medial lemniscus courses along the ventral border of the lateral lemniscus. Its location in the cross-section of the upper part of the midbrain is indicated.

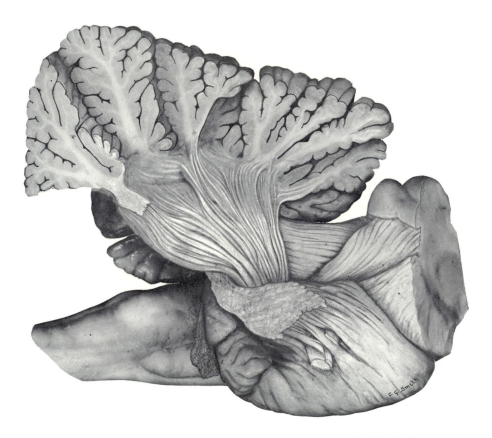

Figure 22a and b. Dissection of the Lateral Aspect of the Cerebellum
Exposing the Radiating Fibers of the Inferior Cerebellar Peduncle.

Dissection

The fibers of the middle cerebellar peduncle were cut dorsal to the fifth cranial nerve
and peeled away to expose the fibers of the
inferior cerebellar peduncle. These fibers
are identifiable by their hook-like course as
they turn into the stalk of the cerebellum
from the medulla. In the process of uncov-
ering the inferior cerebellar peduncle, the
lobules of the inferior surface of the cerebellar hemisphere were removed exposing
the pyramis and the uvula of the vermis.

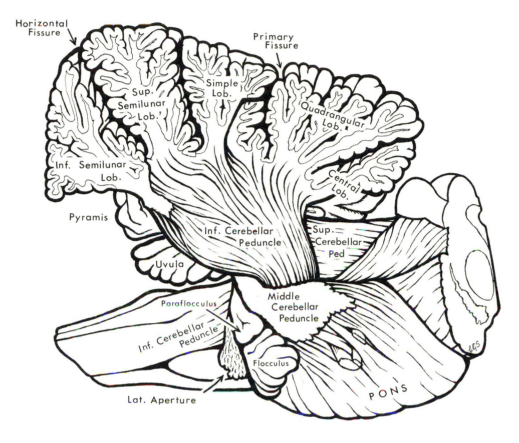

Figure 22b.

Observations

1. The fibers of the inferior cerebellar peduncle form a layer immediately deep to the fibers of the middle cerebellar peduncle. Both peduncles send fibers into each lobule of the cerebellum.
2. The paraflocculus is the lateral portion of a subdivision of the cerebellum that includes the uvula of the vermis and the tonsil of the medial part of the inferior surface of the hemisphere.
3. The lateral aperture of the fourth ventricle is at the end of a sleeve-like extension of its membranous roof. The opening is directed ventrally (see Figure 2).

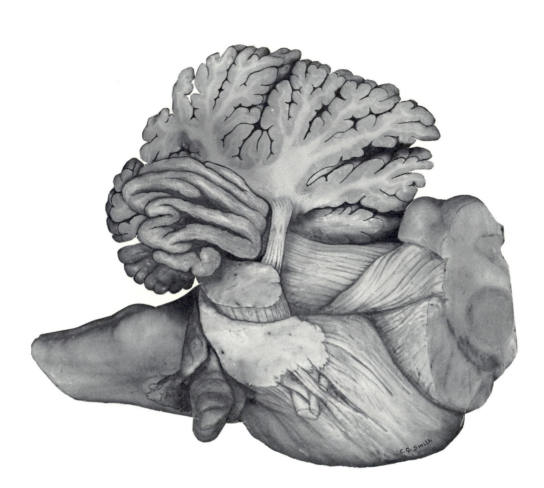

Figure 23a and b. Dissection of the Lateral Aspect of the Cerebellum exposing the Dentate Nucleus, the Superior Cerebellar Peduncle, the Fastigiobulbar Tract and the Uncinate Fasciculus.

Dissection

The fibers of the inferior cerebellar peduncle were cut a short distance dorsal to the previously sectioned middle peduncle and peeled away until the gray matter of the dentate nucleus could be seen. The dentate nucleus was then completely uncovered by removing the thin layer of fibers coming to it from the cerebellar cortex. When this was done, its deep longitudinal furrows were revealed. In carrying out this dissection all the lobules of the hemisphere were removed.

Observations

1. The fibers of the superior cerebellar peduncle emerge from the dentate nucleus.

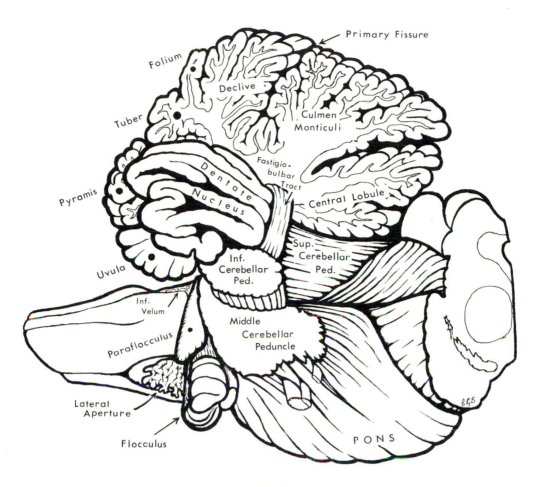

Figure 23b.

2. The bundle of fibers crossing the superior peduncle just rostral to the dentate nucleus is the fastigiobulbar tract. This is an efferent fiber bundle that has its origin in the fastigial nucleus in the vermis. It forms part of the inferior peduncle.

3. Each of the lobules of the cerebellar hemisphere is connected with a lobule of the vermis. The central lobule is connected with the lobule of the same name in the vermis; the quadrangular with the culmen monticuli; the simple lobule with the declive; the superior semilunar with the folium; the inferior semilunar with the tuber; the gracilis lobule with two lobules of the vermis (the tuber and the pyramis); and the biventral with the pyramis. The paraflocculus is connected with the tonsil of the hemisphere and this in turn is connected with the uvula. The flocculus is connected by a slender stalk with the nodule of the vermis.

Section VI

The Major Pathways of the Brain Stem

The Medial Lemniscus

This fiber bundle conveys impulses that excite touch sensation and awareness of position of the parts of the body. It is deep to the surface of the brain except for a brief appearance on the lateral surface of the midbrain. In figure 24 the whole length of the ribbon-like medial lemniscus is isolated in the left half of the brain stem.

The Auditory Pathway

This is the sensory pathway for hearing. It is superficial except for its course in the pons segment. It can be traced, by dissection, into the internal capsule and into the sensory area of cortex in the transverse temporal gyrus. (See Figures 5 and 6.).

The Spinal Tract of the Trigeminal Nerve

This conveys impulses from the sense organs for pain and temperature in the head. Its fibers have their cell bodies in the trigeminal ganglion. It is accessible to the surgeon where it comes to the surface of the medulla.

The Dento-rubro-thalamic Pathway

This pathway conveys impulses from the cerebellum to the cerebral cortex via a relay station in the ventral lateral nucleus of the thalamus. This preparation also provides a partial view of 1) the spiralling medial lemniscus; 2) the pyramidal tract; and 3) the pathway to the anterior nucleus of the thalamus via the fornix, the mammillary body and the mammillo-thalamic tract.

The Optic Pathway

A lesion of this pathway leads to loss of vision. Where the fibers of this pathway are widely separated, as in the optic radiation, a lesion can lead to partial loss of the visual field. A partial loss of vision may also result from pressure on the optic chiasma by a tumor of the pituitary gland.

The Pyramidal Pathway

This is the pathway for voluntary movement. It descends from the precentral gyrus (Figure 4), through the posterior limb of the internal capsule (Figure 16), the crus cerebri of the midbrain, the basilar part of the pons segment (Figure 35), and the pyramid, to decussate as it enters the cord (Figure 27).

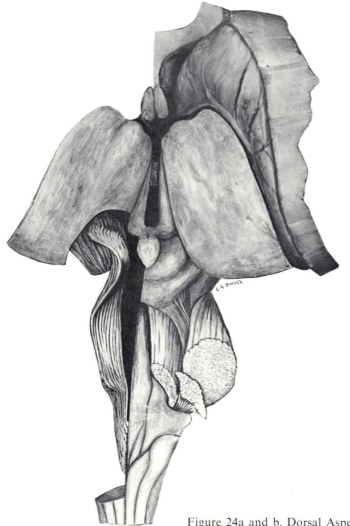

Figure 24a and b. Dorsal Aspect of the Brain Stem.

Dissection

Dissected to expose the medial lemniscus of the left side.

Observations

The ribbon-like medial lemniscus is made up of fibers that have cell bodies in the nucleus gracilis and the nucleus cuneatus, and extend to the posterior ventral lateral nucleus of the diencephalon on the opposite side. Some of its fibers carry impulses from sense organs for touch, others from position-sense organs. These impulses are relayed to the postcentral gyrus of the cerebral hemisphere via the posterior limb of the internal capsule. The nucleus gracilis and the nucleus cuneatus relay impulses from the lower and upper parts of the body respectively.

The medial lemniscus retains its ribbon-like form throughout its length. In the pons the "ribbon" is applied to the dorsal surface of the ventral or basilar part of the pons which contains the pontine nuclei (Figure

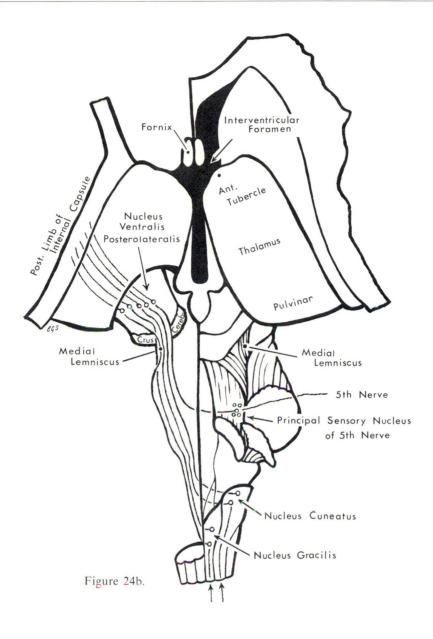

Figure 24b.

35). Here its lateral fibers carry impulses from the leg and lower trunk, the medial fibers convey impulses from the upper trunk and arm. As it enters the midbrain, it shifts laterally into a parasagittal plane where part of it appears on the lateral surface between the brachium of the inferior colliculus and the crus cerebri (Figure 21). As it enters the diencephalon the medial lemniscus "untwists" somewhat so that pathways from the lower trunk and leg are lateral to those from the upper trunk and arm. The pathways for touch and position-

sense from the head are in turn medial to those from the arm. The latter enter the brain in the trigeminal nerve, have a relay station in the principal sensory nucleus of that nerve, and cross the midline to ascend close to the medial border of the medial lemniscus.

The pathways from the leg, the arm, and the head have relay stations in the lateral, the intermediate, and the medial parts of the posterior ventral lateral nucleus, respectively.

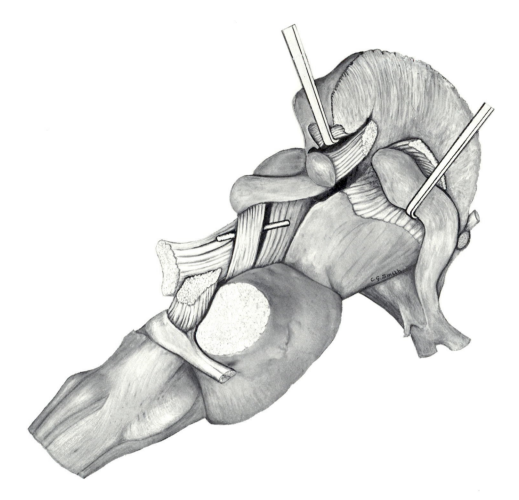

Figure 25a and b. The Auditory Pathway.

Dissection

Dissected to expose the lateral aspect of the brain stem.

Observations

1. The dorsal cochlear nucleus is one of the first relay stations in the auditory pathway to the cerebral cortex.
2. The ribbon-like lateral lemniscus contains fibers of pathways from both the right and the left dorsal cochlear nuclei. The homolateral pathways have an ad-

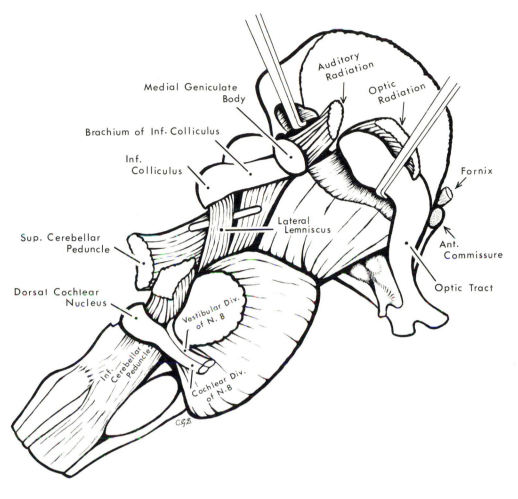

Figure 25b.

ditional relay station in the superior olivary nucleus (Figure 35).

3. The inferior colliculus relays impulses
   via fibers of its brachium to the medial
   geniculate body, a nucleus of the diencephalon. This nucleus relays them in
   turn to the cerebral cortex via the auditory radiation, a part of the internal capsule. In this dissection the optic tract, the

lateral geniculate body, and the optic
radiation have been displaced to expose
the origin of the auditory radiation.

4. Note that cutting the cochlear nerve will
   lead to deafness in one ear, but cutting
   the lateral lemniscus will not seriously
   impair hearing in either ear.

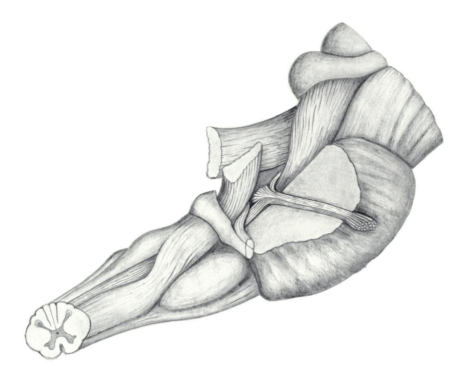

Figure 26a and b. The Spinal Tract of the Trigeminal Nerve.

Dissection

The lateral aspect of the brain stem is dissected as described under observations.

Observations

The spinal tract of the trigeminal nerve (N.5) is a portion of that nerve that descends within the brain stem to end in an elongated nucleus in the caudal part of the medulla and the first cervical segment. This nucleus is called the nucleus of the spinal tract. Its fibers carry impulses from sense organs for pain and changes in temperature. The fibers from the sense organs for touch and the position-sense form a second large bundle that ends in the principal sensory nucleus in the dorsal part of the pons close to the entering fifth nerve. A third small bundle of fibers ascends into the midbrain as the mesencephalic tract of the fifth nerve. This portion of the nerve is atypical in that its fibers have their cell bodies in the

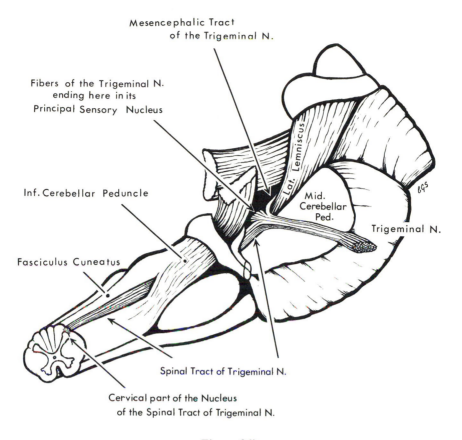

Mesencephalic Tract
of the Trigeminal N.

Fibers of the Trigeminal N.
ending here in its
Principal Sensory Nucleus

Inf. Cerebellar Peduncle

Fasciculus Cuneatus

Lat. Lemniscus

Mid.
Cerebellar
Ped.

Trigeminal N.

Spinal Tract of Trigeminal N.

Cervical part of the Nucleus
of the Spinal Tract of Trigeminal N.

Figure 26b.

midbrain, not in the trigeminal ganglion. The fibers carry impulses from muscle spindles that mediate the stretch reflex, e.g. the jaw jerk.

In Figure 26 the sensory root of the fifth nerve was exposed by cutting across the fibers of the middle cerebellar peduncle at the level of the entering nerve and peeling them away. At the deep border of the peduncle the fibers of the spinal tract were then followed to where they passed deep to the inferior cerebellar peduncle which is embraced by the cochlear and vestibular divisions of the eighth nerve. The spinal tract was then isolated in the lower half of the medulla where it comes to the surface between the fasciculus cuneatus and the fibers of the lateral funiculus that are ascending to form part of the inferior cerebellar peduncle. The fibers of the spinal tract end progressively as it descends and its nucleus gets smaller. At the level of the first cervical segment the nucleus forms the apical portion of the dorsal horn.

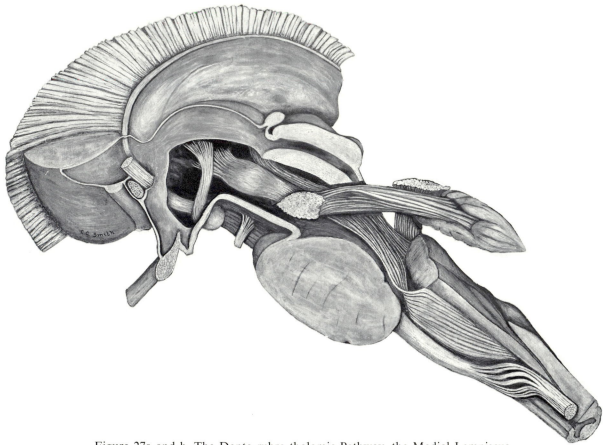

Figure 27a and b. The Dento-rubro-thalamic Pathway, the Medial Lemniscus, and a Portion of the Pyramidal Pathway.

Dissection

A dissection of the medial aspect of the right half of the brain stem.

Observations

1. The dento-rubro-thalamic pathway is a part of the pathway from the cerebellum to the cerebral hemisphere. The nerve fibers (axons) of Purkinje cells in the cerebellar cortex converge on, and synapse in the dentate nucleus. From this sac-like nucleus, in the core of the cerebellum, impulses are relayed along fibers of the superior cerebellar peduncle to the red nucleus of the opposite side.

The superior cerebellar peduncle enters the back of the brain stem medial to the lateral lemniscus and crosses the midline at the level of the inferior colliculus, decussating with its fellow of the opposite side. Having crossed the midline, some of its fibers synapse in the red nucleus which is an ovoid mass located partly in the upper midbrain and partly in the subthalamus of the diencephalon. Some fibers of the superior cerebellar peduncle bypass the red nucleus and ascend together with fibers from the red nucleus to end in the lateral ventral nucleus of the thalamus. In the terminal part of their course they pass lateral to the mammillothalamic fasciculus.

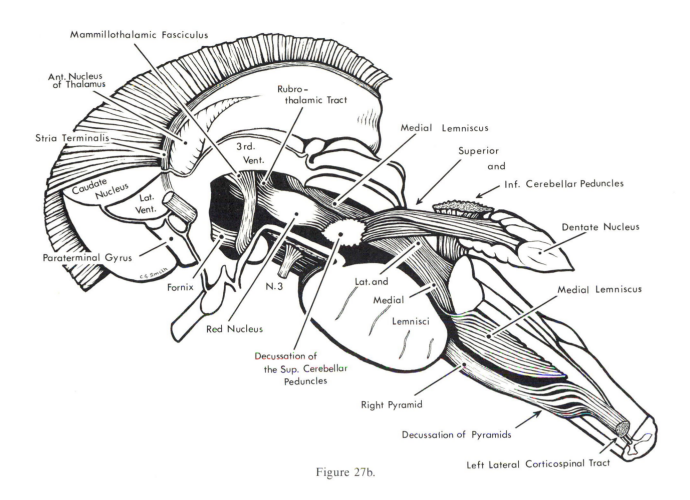

Figure 27b.

2. The medial lemniscus, in this dissection of the right half of the brain stem, is made up of fibers that come from cell bodies of the nuclei gracilis and cuneatus of the left side. In the medulla these fibers form a ribbon-like band in the parasagittal plane just to the right of the median plane. Its ventral border is related to the right pyramid. As it ascends, the ribbon rotates to apply itself to the dorsal surface of the portion of the pons that contains the pontine nuclei. Here it is immediately medial to the lateral lemniscus. In the midbrain it continues its rotation and reaches the lateral surface to lie in a parasagittal plane lateral to the red nucleus. It ends in the posterior ventral lateral nucleus of the diencephalon just caudal to the termination of the rubrothalamic tract.

3. The pyramidal tract emerges from the pons to form the external feature of the medulla called the pyramid. Most of the fibers of the pyramid cross the midline in the caudal quarter of the medulla to form the lateral corticospinal tract. This tract is located in the lateral funiculus immediately lateral to the dorsal horn. The fibers that do not cross have not been isolated. They continue into the medial part of the ventral funiculus of the same side.

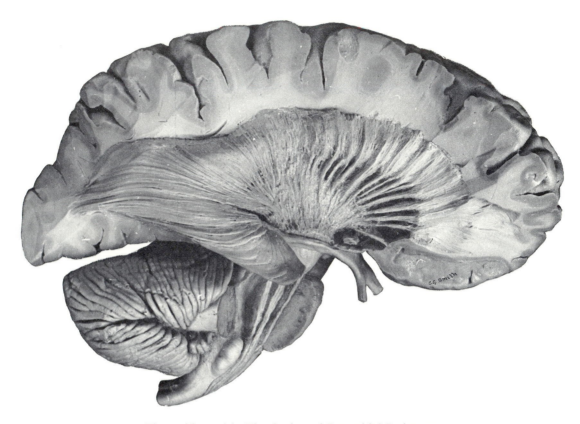

Figure 28a and b. The Optic and Pyramidal Pathways.

Dissections

A dissection of the lateral aspect of the whole brain.

Observations

The Optic Pathway

The optic nerve is attached to the anterior end of the diencephalon. Here the fibers of the nasal half of each eye separate from the fibers of the temporal half to decussate in the floor of the third ventricle and form the optic chiasma. The temporal fibers are joined by the nasal fibers from the eye of the opposite side to form the optic tract. This tract crosses the crus cerebri just below the attachment of the hemisphere to the diencephalon and extends to the lateral geniculate body located on the inferior surface of the pulvinar.

The fibers of the cells in the lateral geniculate body make up the optic radiation and enter the sublenticular part of the internal capsule to fan out in the wall of the lateral ventricle and reach the visual sensory cortex. This cortex is located in the walls of the posterior part of the calcarine sulcus on the medial surface of the occipital lobe. In this preparation the fibers of the optic radiation were isolated from the other fibers of the internal capsule by passing a hook around the optic tract to free it and lift it and the lateral geniculate body, with its outgoing fibers, from its bed.

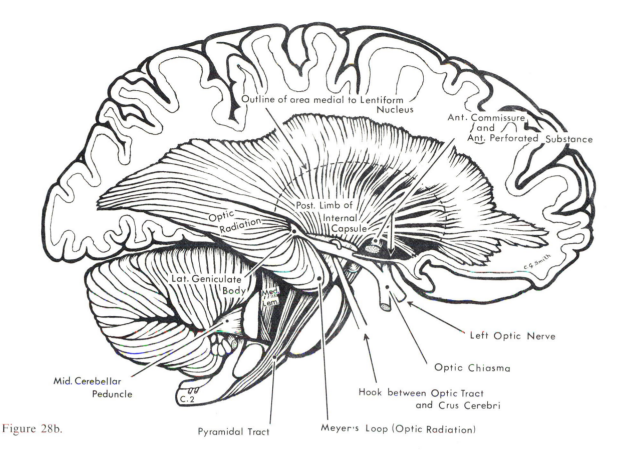

Figure 28b.

The fibers of the optic radiation form a thin ribbon-like band about 2 cm wide. The upper fibers course almost directly backward, but the lower fibers curve progressively toward the temporal pole before looping backward. This is clinically significant because injuries to the temporal pole may involve these fibers, known as Meyer's loop. The result is loss of vision in the lower homolateral quadrants of both eyes.

The Pyramidal Tract

The fibers of the pyramidal tract descend in the corona radiata and in the posterior limb of the internal capsule. They are joined by fibers of the corticopontine tracts to form the crus cerebri which plunges into the ven-

tral part of the pons. There the corticopontine fibers synapse with cells of the pontine nucleus. These cells relay impulses along fibers which cross the midline to form the middle cerebellar peduncle. The fibers of the pyramidal tract are in several bundles that pass through the pontine nucleus without interruption. They come together to form a compact bundle as they reach the medulla where they form the pyramid. In this preparation the fiber bundles of the pyramidal tract were exposed in the pons by following them up from the medulla to the crus cerebri.

Section VII

Stained Sections of the Brain

1. Figures 29, 30, and 31 show slices of the whole brain stained with nigrosin. This technique stains the gray matter black and leaves the white matter unstained.
2. Figures 32, 33, 34, 35, 36, and 37, show sections of the brain stem stained using the Weigert technique. This method stains the white matter black and leaves the gray matter unstained.

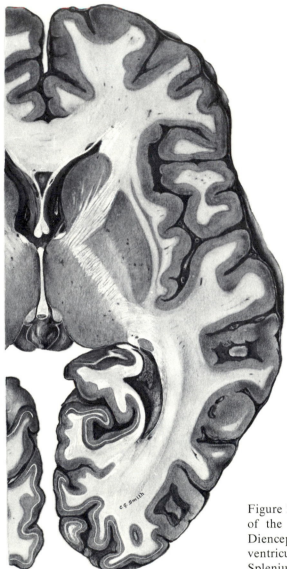

Figure 29a and b. A Horizontal Section of the Cerebral Hemisphere and the Diencephalon at the Level of the Interventricular Foramen and Inferior to the Splenium of the Corpus Callosum.

Observations

1. The cortex of the visual sensory area is identified by a white line called the line of Gennari. This is a layer of fibers, i.e. the myelinated terminals of the optic radiation.
2. The fornix is sectioned posteriorly where it forms a fringe-like band at the border of the hippocampus, and also anteriorly where it forms the inferior border of the septum pellucidum.
3. The cavity in the septum pellucidum does not communicate with the ventricular system.
4. The anterior part of the internal capsule between the caudate nucleus and the lentiform nucleus is the anterior limb.

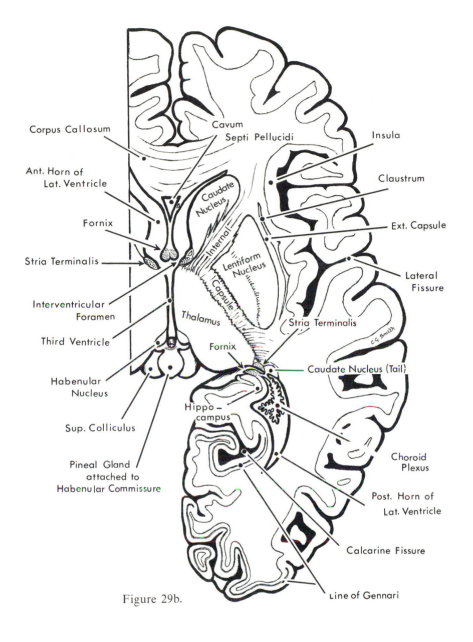

Figure 29b.

Corpus Callosum

Ant. Horn of
Lat. Ventricle

Fornix

Stria Terminalis

Interventricular
Foramen

Third Ventricle

Habenular
Nucleus

Sup. Colliculus

Pineal Gland
attached to
Habenular Commissure

Cavum
Septi Pellucidi

Caudate
Nucleus

Internal

Lentiform
Nucleus

Capsule

Thalamus

Fornix

Hippo –
campus

Insula

Claustrum

Ext. Capsule

Lateral
Fissure

Stria Terminalis

Caudate Nucleus (Tail)

Choroid
Plexus

Post. Horn of
Lat. Ventricle

Calcarine Fissure

Line of Gennari

C.G. Smith

Here the fibers are cut lengthwise. The knee-like bend in the internal capsule is the genu. The posterior limb lies between the thalamus of the diencephalon and the lentiform nucleus. The portion of the posterior limb posterior to the lentiform nucleus is called the retrolentiform part. The tail of the caudate nucleus is medial to it.

5. The pale medial segment of the lentiform nucleus is called the globus pallidus. Its lateral portion is the putamen.

6. The insula forms the floor of the lateral fissure.

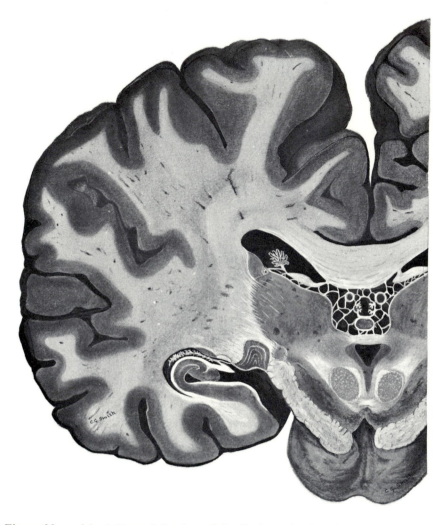

Figure 30a and b. A Frontal Section of the Brain at the Level of the Junction of
the Midbrain and the Diencephalon.

Observations

1. The posterior commissure is part of the light reflex pathway. Its fibers convey impulses from one eye to excite constriction of the pupil of the opposite eye.
2. The pineal recess is an extension of the third ventricle into the stalk of the pineal gland. The suprapineal recess is a pouch-like diverticulum of the roof of the third ventricle that extends back above the pineal gland (see Figure 14).
3. The cells of the lateral geniculate body, a relay station of the optic pathway, are arranged in layers like those of the retina and the visual cortex.
4. The stria terminalis and the caudate nucleus encircle the attachment of the

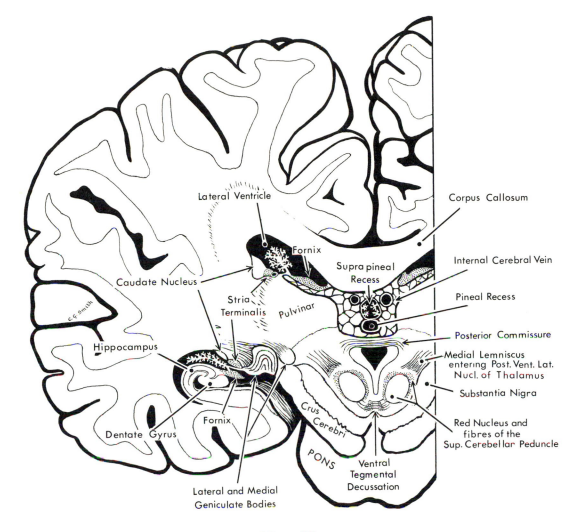

Figure 30b.

hemisphere to the diencephalon. Therefore, both are cut twice, once in the section of the inferior horn and a second time in the section of the body of the lateral ventricle. The stria terminalis extends from the amygdaloid nucleus, at the tip of the inferior horn, to the interventricular foramen where it enters the hypothalamus lateral to the fornix.

5. The fornix is the efferent fiber bundle of the hippocampus. It has an arched course (see Figure 13) and is cut twice in this frontal section, once at its origin in the inferior horn and again where it forms part of the wall of the body of the lateral ventricle.

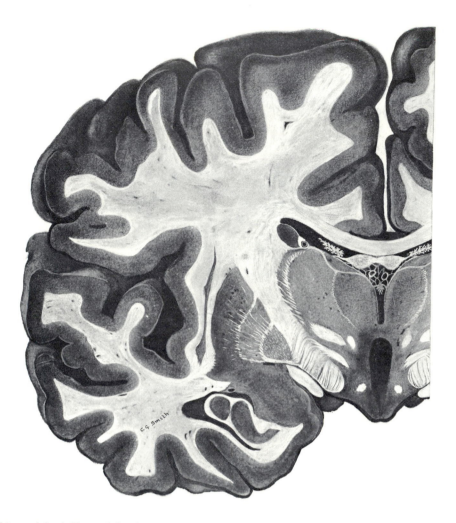

Figure 31a and b. A Frontal Section of the Brain at the Level of the Middle of the Diencephalon.

Observations

1. The lenticular fasciculus is an efferent pathway of the globus pallidus. Its fibers penetrate the internal capsule to reach the subthalamus just anterior to the red nucleus. Here some fibers turn dorsally and anteriorly to join fibers of the rubrothalamic tract to form the thalamic fasciculus.

2. The thalamic fasciculus is sectioned just ventral to the lateral ventral nucleus of the thalamus where some of its fibers end. Its remaining fibers end, anterior to this level, in the anterior ventral lateral nucleus.

3. The mammillothalamic fasciculus is cut across as it arches dorsally from the mammillary body to reach the anterior nucleus of the thalamus. Impulses are relayed by the anterior nucleus to the cortex of the limbic lobe that influence emotional feeling.

4. The Adhesio Interthalamica is aptly called an adhesion. It is a band of gray matter that connects the right and left medial thalamic nuclei. It is large in most mammals, but in the human brain

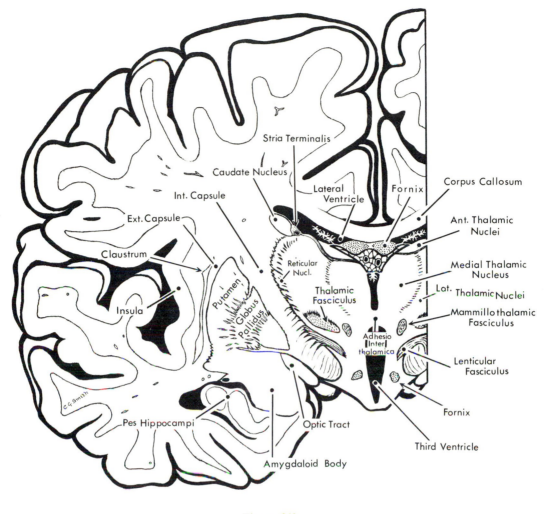

Figure 31b.

it varies in size and was absent in 14 of 52 brains examined by the author.

5. The medial and lateral thalamic nuclei are separated by a thin layer of loosely disposed myelinated fibers called the internal medullary lamina (not labeled). Within this lamina are the cells of the intralaminar nuclei, a part of the medial thalamus. Caudal to the level of this section the lamina encloses a large nucleus of this group called the centromedian nucleus.

6. The fibers leaving the lateral side of the lateral thalamic nuclei pass through a thin outer layer of cells, the reticular nucleus of the thalamus.

7. The globus pallidus is divided into inner and outer segments.

8. The pes hippocampi is the broad anterior end of the hippocampal eminence. Its name reflects its resemblance to an animal's paw (see Figure 10).

9. The fornix is cut twice, once below the corpus callosum and again within the diencephalon, where it courses posteriorly to end in the mammillary body of the hypothalamus.

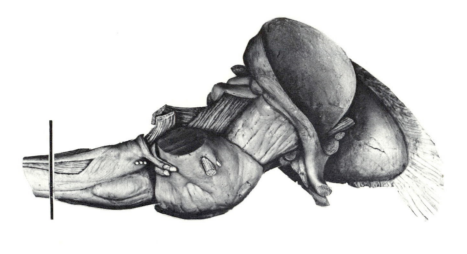

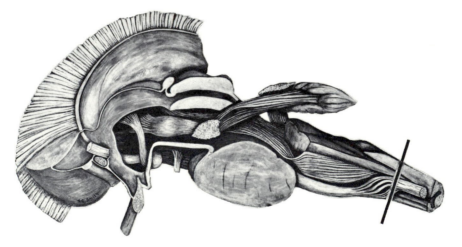

Figure 32a and b.

Observations

1. The fibers of the lateral corticospinal tract cross the midline obliquely. In this section they have begun to shift medially and ventrally from their position in the lateral funiculus and have reached the midline. In passing through the gray matter, they isolate the ventral horn.

2. The section passes through the caudal end of the nucleus gracilis and the nucleus cuneatus. The latter is just beginning to invade the fasciculus cuneatus.

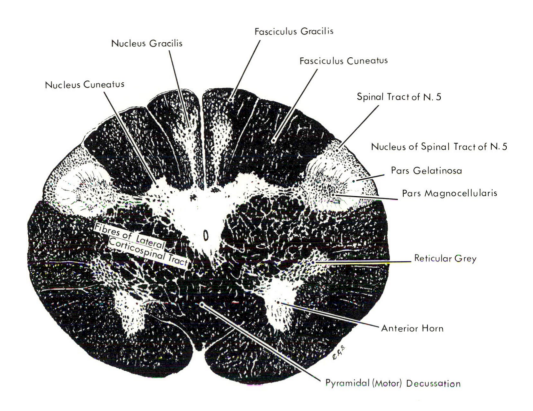

Figure 32a, b and c. A Cross-section of the Medulla Oblongata
Through the Caudal Part of the Motor Decussation
(the plane of the section is indicated in
Figure 32a and 32b).

These nuclei are relay stations for the sensory pathways of the posterior funiculus. The pathways in the fasciculus gracilis enter the cord below the mid-thoracic region; those in the fasciculus cuneatus enter the cord above that level.

3. The gray matter at the tip of the posterior horn is the sensory nucleus of the spinal tract of the fifth cranial nerve. The fibers of this tract are thinly myelinated. They carry impulses from pain and temperature sense organs.

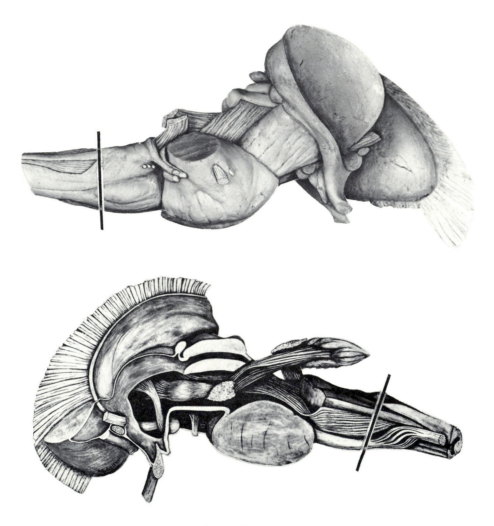

Figure 33a and b.

Observations

1. The fasciculus gracilis and cuneatus get progressively smaller as their fibers drop out to end in their respective nuclei.
2. The cells of the nucleus gracilis and cuneatus give rise to internal arcuate fibers that arch ventrally and medially to cross the midline and ascend in a ribbon-like bundle called the medial lemniscus.
3. The pyramid contains the fibers of the corticospinal tracts. Arterioles that supply the pyramid also supply the medial lemniscus. Hence, occlusion of these vessels will result in paralysis and loss of touch and position senses on the opposite side of the body.

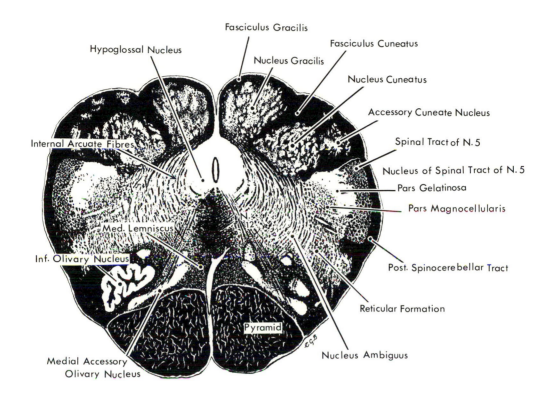

Figure 33a, b and c. A Section of the Medulla Oblongata
Showing the Decussation of the Sensory Pathways that
Ascend in the Posterior Funiculi of the Spinal cord
(See Figure 33a and 33b for the plane of the section).

4. The sensory nuclei that form the posterior horn of the cord are represented here by the nuclei gracilis, cuneatus, and the nucleus of the spinal tract of the fifth nerve. The motor nucleus of the hypoglossal nerve is located ventrolateral to the central canal. The motor nucleus of the vagus (a part of the nucleus ambiguus) is located in the central part of each half of the section. The rest of the gray matter is comparable to the intermediate gray of the cord. It includes the reticular gray and the nuclei of the olivary complex. The latter are important relay nuclei on pathways to the cerebellum.

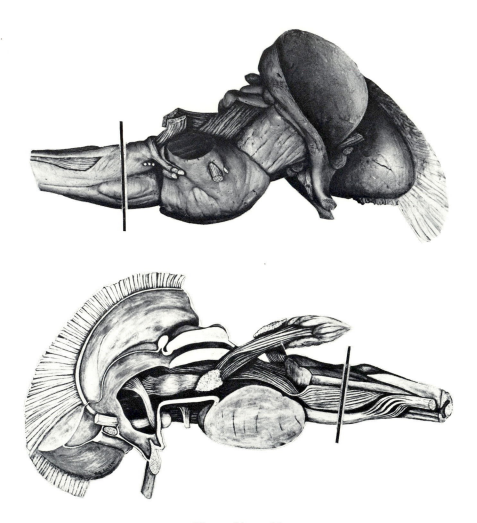

Figure 34a and b.

Observations

The lateral and ventral corticospinal tracts are together in the pyramid. The pathways of the fasciculi gracilis and cuneatus have decussated and are together in the medial lemniscus. The central canal has enlarged to form the fourth ventricle and the dorsal wall of the neural tube is reduced to a thin membrane called the inferior velum. The midline opening in this membrane is the median aperture (Foramen of Magendie) through which cerebrospinal fluid escapes into the subarachnoid space. The choroid plexus of the fourth ventricle is prolonged backward to form the tufted border of this aperture.

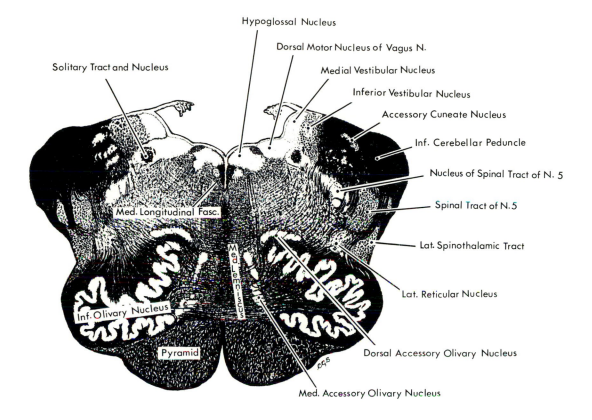

Figure 34a, b and c. A Section of the Medulla Oblongata Through
the Caudal Part of the Fourth Ventricle. (The plane
of the section is indicated in Figure 34a and 34b).

Motor and sensory nuclei are found in the floor of the fourth ventricle. These correspond to the nuclei of the anterior and posterior horns of the cord. The nucleus of the solitary tract is the visceral sensory (e.g., taste) nucleus of the seventh, ninth, and tenth cranial nerves. The fibers of these nerves make up the solitary tract. The nucleus of the spinal tract of the fifth cranial nerve is separated from its tract by olivo-cerebellar fibers that form a major part of the inferior cerebellar peduncle.

The medial longitudinal fasciculus is a bundle of fibers that have their origin in the vestibular nuclei and extend to motor nuclei involved in righting balance reflexes. Some are ascending and some are descending.

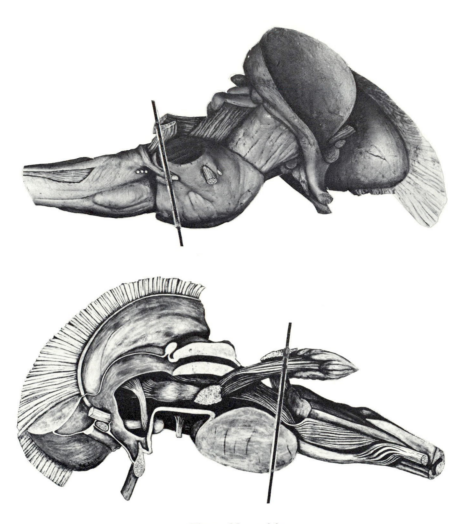

Figure 35a and b.

Observations

The pons segment has dorsal and ventral parts. The ventral part contains the pontine nuclei. These nuclei are relay stations on a pathway from the cerebral cortex to the cerebellum. The cells of these nuclei give rise to fibers that cross the midline to form the middle cerebellar peduncle. The pyramidal tract passes through the pontine nuclei without interruption.

The dorsal part of the pons segment forms the floor of the fourth ventricle, is covered on its lateral side by the middle cerebellar peduncle, and has the medial lemniscus in its ventral border. The medial lemniscus is penetrated by fibers of the auditory pathway that cross the midline to ascend lateral to the superior olivary nucleus and form the ribbon-like bundle called the lateral lemniscus. The superior olivary nucleus is a relay station on a homolateral auditory pathway. Fibers of this nucleus join the lateral lemniscus.

The nucleus of the abducent nerve (N.6) is close to the midline in the floor of the

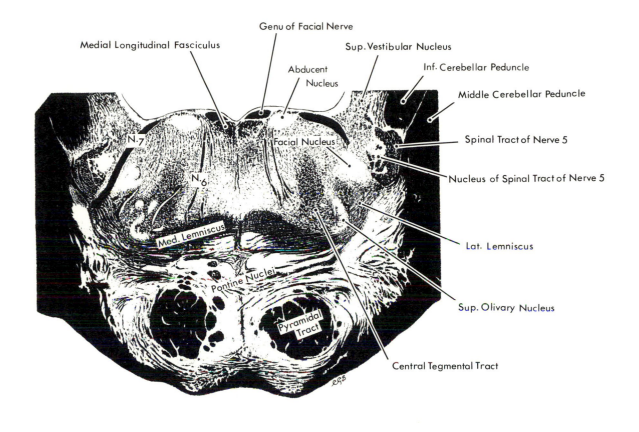

Genu of Facial Nerve

Medial Longitudinal Fasciculus

Sup. Vestibular Nucleus

Abducent
Nucleus

Inf. Cerebellar Peduncle

Middle Cerebellar Peduncle

N.7

Facial Nucleus

Spinal Tract of Nerve 5

N.6

Nucleus of Spinal Tract of Nerve 5

Med. Lemniscus

Lat. Lemniscus

Pontine Nuclei

Pyramidal
Tract

Sup. Olivary Nucleus

Central Tegmental Tract

Figure 35a, b and c. A Cross-section of the Pons Segment at the Level Indicated in Figure 35a and 35b.

fourth ventricle. Its fibers course ventrally *and* caudally to their point of exit from the brain stem; therefore, only a part of this nerve is present in this cross-section. The nucleus of the facial nerve (N.7) is located dorsal to the superior olivary nucleus. Its fibers loop around the nucleus of the sixth nerve to form an elevation in the floor of the fourth ventricle called the facial colliculus. From here the seventh nerve courses ventrally and caudally between its own nucleus and the nucleus of the spinal tract of nerve 5 (sensory).

The central tegmental tract conveys impulses from the red nucleus and other parts of the upper midbrain to the inferior olivary nucleus in the medulla oblongata. This tract also contains reticulothalamic fibers. The medial longitudinal fasciculus conveys impulses from the vestibular nuclei to motor nuclei at higher and lower levels.

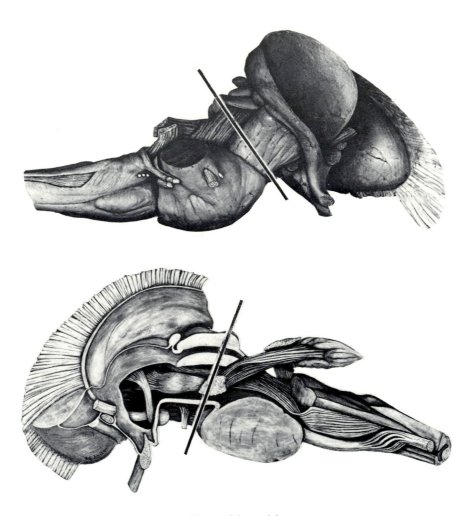

Figure 36a and b.

Observations

The identifying features of this level of the midbrain are the nuclei of the inferior colliculi and the decussating fibers of the superior cerebellar peduncles. The inferior colliculi are relay stations on the auditory pathway to the cerebral cortex. They are partially encapsulated by the terminating fibers of the lateral lemniscus. The inferior colliculus also gives rise to fibers of the tectospinal tract that course ventrally and cross the midline dorsal to the decussation of the superior cerebellar peduncles. Having crossed, they descend ventral to the medial longitudinal fasciculus to reach the motor nuclei of the brain stem and the spinal cord. They mediate reflex responses such as head turning. In this preparation the descending fibers are obscured by decussating fibers.

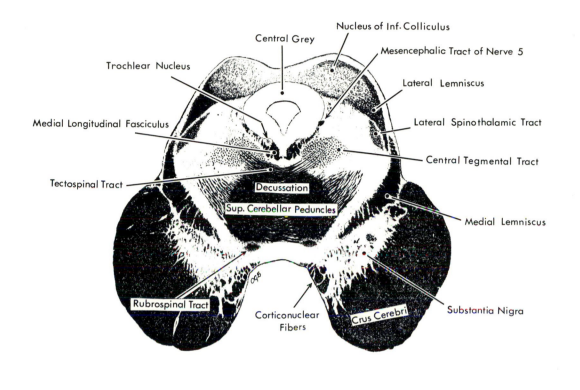

Figure 36a, b and c. A Section of the Lower Part of the
Midbrain at the Level Indicated in
Figure 36a and 36b.

The small trochlear nucleus (N.4), in the ventral part of the central gray, is partly surrounded by fibers of the medial longitudinal fasciculus some of which end in it. Lateral to the central gray is the slender mesencephalic tract of the fifth nerve. Cell bodies of these fibers are located in the lateral part of the central gray matter.

The crus cerebri contains the corticopontine and pyramidal tracts. The substantia nigra, a layer of pigmented cells, intervenes between the crus cerebri and the medial part of the medial lemniscus. The pigment is washed out of these cells in the process of staining the section. The central tegmental tract is poorly defined and at this level most of its fibers are reticulothalamic. Corticonuclear corticobulbar fibers are pyramidal tract fibers that end in the motor nuclei of the pons and the medulla oblongata.

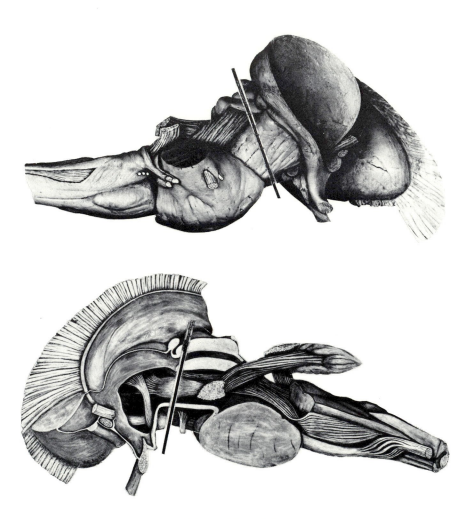

Figure 37a and b.

Observations

The identifying features of this section are the red nuclei and the laminated gray matter of the superior colliculi.

The superior colliculus receives impulses from the visual cortex of the cerebral hemisphere via the striatum opticum, and impulses conveyed by the medial lemniscus via the stratum lemnisci. The superior colliculus mediates postural changes via efferent fibers that form the stratum profundum. They course ventrally around the central gray to cross the midline and descend just ventral to the medial longitudinal fasciculus. These are fibers of the tectospinal tract.

The substantia nigra is coextensive with the deep surface of the crus cerebri. It receives afferents from the globus pallidus (pallidonigral tract) and gives rise to efferents that ascend to the striatum (nigrostriate tract).

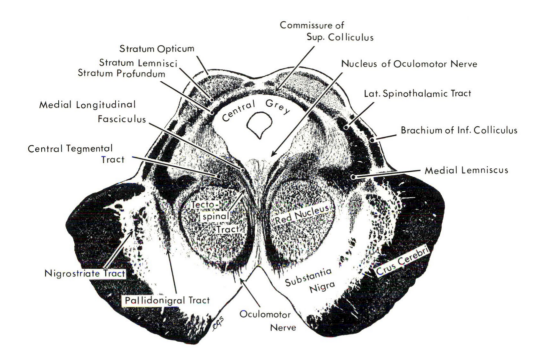

Figure 37a, b and c. A Section of the Upper Part of the
Midbrain at the Level Indicated in
Figure 37a and 37b.

The brachium of the inferior colliculus relays auditory impulses from the inferior colliculus to the medial geniculate body of the diencephalon. The lateral spinothalamic tract is deep to the brachium where it may be cut to relieve pain on the opposite side of the body. Cutting the overlying brachium does not significantly impair hearing because there is a pathway to both hemispheres from each ear.

The ventral part of the central gray contains the nuclei of the oculomotor nerve. Fibers of this nerve penetrate the red nucleus to emerge at the medial border of the crus cerebri. The central tegmental tract, at this level, contains reticulothalamic fibers and some descending fibers from the corpus striatum that will be joined by fibers from the red nucleus to end in the inferior olivary nucleus.

Index

References are to Figure Numbers